# The Colic Manual: Redefining What Colic Is and How to Treat It

By Dennis Scharenberg, D.C.

Cover Design: Matthew Cropsey and Krystahl Goodale
Picture by: Emily Southerland
Pictures throughout book were used with permission of families and
photographers
Graphic in Ch. 7 by: Melissa

Copyright © 2016 Dennis Scharenberg, D.C.
**www.stoppingcolic.com**

ISBN: 0692791922

ISBN-13: 978-0692791929

# Table of Content

# Preface

This colic manual was not written to make doctors out of parents. This manual was written to give as many parents as possible an understanding of the condition that has plagued mankind since the beginning. Since the beginning of man, babies have cried and parents have tried everything they could think of to get them to stop crying! Crying is something that is very hard to tolerate because it carries with it so many emotions--fear, pain, sadness, happiness, anger, love, loneliness, hunger, fatigue, anxiety, rejection, and anticipation.

When adults cry, you can ask them why. Babies are different. They cannot speak to you in a language that you can understand with words. They are only concerned with how they are feeling. Because babies cannot talk to us and tell us what is making them uncomfortable, we as parents or caregivers have to guess what is wrong.

My lifetime of research has shown me that we have not come very far in understanding what babies are trying to tell us when they cry. Most current research claims that it is simply common for all babies to cry and fuss and that crying is just a part of being a baby. I disagree.

My research indicates that approximately 95% of babies do not have a pathological problem that is causing them to cry. They are crying because of something that is making them uncomfortable or something that can be corrected without medical attention such as drugs or surgery.

It is true that babies do get sick. They can get sinus infections, ear infections, bronchial infections, and pneumonia, as well as certain conditions, such as failing to thrive, and genetic conditions such as Williams's disease and birth defects. Most newborns, however, are generally born healthy in the United States and other technologically advanced countries. There are many exceptions in economically deprived countries, where poor nourishment and health care is limited.

This book was written with the intention of helping the reader better understand why our babies cry and how to deal with colic, which has caused thousands and thousands of parents heartache. This heartache is mostly due because babies cry most commonly in the first few months of their lives, and there doesn't seem to be an answer to successfully explain, treat, and prevent this painful condition known as colic. Through this book, I would like to show you what I have researched and discovered in the last forty years about colic, how I would redefine colic, the true cause of colic, and I would like to explain my technique, which I have used and continue to use every day to counter colic. My goal for the future is not only to help the babies who are suffering from colic symptoms, but, eventually, to prevent colic all together.

I realize there are testimonials from all facets of medical, chiropractic, and homeopathic professions that have helped in certain colic cases; however, I could not find recent or continuing studies to prove that colic could be corrected consistently with any of these remedies or techniques. I believe that my technique, which eases a baby's colic, while creating no side effects or harm, is worth considering.

No one will be more motivated to treat and spend the time necessary to treat their baby's colic than a mother or father. The person treating the baby must have a sincere desire to stick with the treatment, while also having the patience to continue this care until the treatment is complete. They must be able to spend enough time and energy on the baby in order to correct this problem, because it is not enough simply to offer a treatment, whether chemical or physical, and hope the baby gets well. The baby will only get well if this treatment is done correctly.

The best way to use this book is to read it from cover to cover. Many themes are repeated to help you, as a reader, see how integral this information is to helping your baby. The better you understand the information, the more you will understand the educational videos that complement this book. There are many advertised shortcuts and bargains for treating colic. This is not a short-cut technique. This is about you, the parent, learning and studying the information I have found to be true in order to get your baby well. I adore babies, and my passion has been finding a way to relieve them of this deadly, awful, and painful condition.

This book is for educational purposes only and is not meant to diagnose or treat. The opinions offered in this book are that of the author based on his experiences of working with thousands of infants and parents.

# Chapter 1: What is Colic?

### *The history and medical explanation of colic*

## My story

In January of 1973, I graduated from college. That March, my wife and I welcomed our first son into the world. A year later, my second son was born. It was the time in my life of beginnings. I was starting a family and a career. I lived in a small town in Kansas, and as I opened my practice, families started bringing screaming babies to me. The babies were in pain, and as a father myself, I understood the desperation in the parents' voices as they asked for help. Parents will move mountains to help their child. And so I started looking into the condition known as colic. Many of the babies coming in had stories similar to the story below. Maybe you can relate as well.

Since the day she found out she was pregnant, Allison started dreaming and counting down the weeks until she would meet her precious baby. She took classes and made baby wish lists. Then, the day came. Allison held her precious little one and couldn't believe how much love she had in her heart. As soon as Allison placed her baby down in the bassinet to sleep, the baby screamed and screamed.

She tried some of the soothing techniques she had learned at her prenatal classes with some success, but after two weeks of hours upon hours of distressed crying, Allison was worried and mentioned the situation to her pediatrician.

"Colic is very common in newborns," he said. Allison was heartbroken. She felt like she was a bad mother. How could she help her baby? She started looking for answers. Article after article said there was no cure for colic. There were plenty of advertisements saying their product would ease colic, but nothing seemed to permanently work.

Allison's mom tried to comfort her, "You were also very colicky. You didn't cry as much after 3 months. It will pass." With fatigue and desperation setting in, Allison wasn't sure she could last that long.

**Medical history of Colic**

This is the reality for many parents, and the sad truth is that the medical community does not have a lot of answers or lasting solutions for babies with colic symptoms. Looking at the history of colic, along with theories and proposed remedies, I will show how colic has been perceived and how there is something wrong with the current colic diagnosis. By the end of the chapter, I will redefine the definition of colic and describe what I have found to be the major cause of colic. But first, the history.

In 1954 pediatrician Dr. Morris Wessel described colic as a baby crying inconsolably for three hours a day, three days per week, for at least three weeks. He stated that the baby would grow out of the colic condition in three months. Dr. Wessel said that no one really knew the cause of colic, and no one knew how to treat the condition successfully. He also stated that it was not a serious health problem since the baby would outgrow it and was not physically sick with anything else.

Today there has been very little change in the diagnosis, treatment, or known cause of colic, even though the medical community estimates that approximately 40% of the baby population has this condition.[1] Although sometimes the symptoms of colic could suggest a more serious ailment, most pediatricians regard it as part of normal infant development.  The use of medication has not been recommended for colic because the risk of harmful side effects outweigh the benefits for an otherwise healthy baby. Instead, doctors may recommend homeopathic remedies. Although these remedies do not seem to cure, they don't create any harmful side effects on the baby. In many cases, they may treat the symptoms temporarily, leaving some relief for babies and caregivers.

Along with homeopathic remedies, various other inventions have been developed to help colicky babies, such as swings, which keep the baby in an elevated position and create motion. Other products include blankets for swaddling or baby carriers for keeping the baby in an upright position. These inventions have in many cases proved helpful in soothing the baby, but it has never proven to treat the condition of colic or to eliminate the underlying cause. These are mainly soothing techniques.

Along with severe crying, there are many other symptoms associated with colic. One symptom doctors can treat is the spit up or projectile vomiting. These colic symptoms are diagnosed as acid reflux. A doctor can prescribe an acid reflux medication such as Zantac, Prilosec, Tegument, etc. to support the acid reflux symptoms. This medication does not usually stop the spit up or the projectile vomiting; however, doctors continue to prescribe medication because it neutralizes the stomach acid and helps prevent burning and erosion of the esophageal tissue. Again, the baby will still continue to spit up.

The current colic theory says that infants should outgrow colic by the end of six months. Many babies do improve as they grow older; however, the condition of poor digestion and abnormal bowel function is still present in some form for many of those babies. Constipation seems to be the most common complaint, and many children end up taking some form of stool softener such as Miralax to keep their bowel movements regular.

Those same children grow into adults who continue to experience digestive problems. Many of the advertisements targeted to adults with digestive problems are very similar to the symptoms of a colicky baby. Colic is common in adults as well as children, and it is also very common in horses. For anyone who has had digestive or abnormal bowel functions, the experience can be painful, inconvenient, and even embarrassing. However, an adult, and even a child in some situations, is able to describe their discomfort to a physician and seek some sort of relief. For a baby, on the other hand, who is unable to communicate except through crying, the experience is excruciating. This is true not only for the baby, but also for the parents and anyone else who is a caregiver to the baby.

## Purple Crying

Unable to offer an explanation or better treatment options to parents has to be devastating to physicians as well. Colic is a serious condition, which causes severe crying, as well as many other symptoms, and creates severe emotional pain to all members of the immediate family. Although the diagnosis and treatment of colic has not changed, the way it is being presented to parents has. In association with the National Center on Shaken Baby Syndrome in the United States, pediatrician Dr. Ronald G. Barr gave infant crying and colic a new name called "Period of PURPLE crying." The message of Purple Crying is an encouragement to parents and caregivers that it is not just 40% of babies who inconsolably cry but that *all* babies cry. Again, there is no explanation given with Purple Crying as to why babies cry beyond the idea that it is a developmental stage that all babies must go through.

This campaign was created in response to the thousands of

babies injured and killed due to Shaken Baby Syndrome. A 2001 report estimates that 1,400 babies die from Shaken Baby Syndrome each year.[2] The basic definition of Shaken Baby Syndrome is that a baby's continued crying and screaming becomes intolerable for a caregiver. This frustration, coupled with fatigue from the constant care that is needed for a new infant and the sleep deprivation that occurs, creates a situation where a caregiver finally reaches a breaking point and shakes or suffocates the baby. Family, friends, significant others, or daycare providers are unintentionally killing these babies because they can no longer continue listening to the uncontrollable crying.

The main message of "Period of PURPLE crying" does not give any solution to treating or curing colic. It only addresses the fact that colic is the main reason for Shaken Baby Syndrome and gives encouragement to caregivers. One of their major pieces of advice is to put the baby in another room, shut the door, walk away, and do something else for 15 minutes before going back to comfort the baby. This gives caregivers a little time to regain their composure so that they will not harm the baby.

Generally, parents do not intentionally want to harm or kill their babies, but there seems to be a breaking point when people can no longer listen to any more crying. Organizations that are trying to prevent harm and death to these babies should be applauded; however, "Period of PURPLE CRYING" does not address the cause of colic or give suggestions on how to relieve it.

The following testimonial demonstrates the seriousness of the condition of colic. Most literature states that you should not to worry about colic. It is supposed to start at 3 weeks and end at 3 months "normally called the rule of 3". My experience over the years indicated this is generally not true. As the baby is born with many of the symptoms of colic and will continue on through life. The diagnosis changes such as calling it colic, acid reflux, and indigestion, IBS, Chrones and many other conditions where the causes seem to be unknown.

My experience indicates that many adults continue on with many digestive problems and these people continue on medication such as Prilosec, Zantac, Tegamet, etc. My opinion is that if colic is not addressed as an infant that many people will continue on with some kind of digestive problem for the remainder of their life.

This testimonial was given by one of the most gentle and caring Christian Man I have ever known. When your child is hurting and crying and you can't do anything to comfort your child the stress is sometimes more than some people can tolerate.

My thanks and appreciation goes out to this patient as even years later he can vividly remember how painful it was. Thank you for being so honest. I know people will appreciate your humbleness in giving this testimonial and that hopefully we can protect their babies from harm.

## **"One Dad's Story"**

The day Dr. S saved my family.

When my first child was born, I thought I nailed it being a father.

What was so hard about this? He slept easily, ate well, barely cried, and had a good disposition. Basically, a great baby. Hey, we got this, I told my wife, let us have another blessing. Then came my daughter...

What a totally different experience she was. Out of the womb, literally, she screamed her head off and we even got a picture of her being weighed, while giving us the "bird" with her hand. Oh boy, I thought, this one is feisty. How correct I was. From the first night, this child screamed her head off. We thought to ourselves, just let it go for a while, it will be ok. Well, it wasn't. My daughter screamed and cried almost continuously night and day. I thought this would go away, but it was incessant. The doctor called it Colic. Said it would go away in 2 or 3 weeks. Nope. We tried altering the wife's diet, all the way down to nothing but cheerios. We saw doctor after doctor. We tried medicines, gas reducing pills, pacifiers, putting her on top of the dryer on spin cycle, driving in the car at different speeds and surfaces,

I mean we tried EVERYTHING. She was fed, held, burped, changed, clean, sang to, rocked, and everything else you could think of. Nothing worked.

Now to put this in context, this happened over weeks and weeks. The only thing that helped was when my wife was breast feeding her, and sometimes, not even that worked. This whole scenario was causing a huge strain on our family. Wife was exhausted, my son was cranky too, and I was irritable. It was the most helpless feeling I have ever had. Why could I not fix this? I grew increasingly angry towards this baby. I started to hate her. I just wanted some peace and quiet in our home. I even tried putting her in the downstairs basement just to get away from the screams. Could hear them plainly through the vents.

I consider myself to be a very stable individual. I have a good education, don't drink, smoke, or do drugs. I have good mental capacity and work a normal job. I have never understood how anyone could possibly hurt a child. Something must be wrong with "those" people. That is why the next part I share makes this so scary. I finally understand how people can snap.

It was around 2am and my daughter had been crying for about 5 or 6 hours straight.  My wife was just plain out exhausted and needed a break.  My son, not quite 2 at the time, was mad and crying too as he couldn't sleep through the screaming either.  I had been at work all day and just wanted to sleep.  The screeching was incessant.  "SHUT THE HELL UP YOU STUPID BABY!" just screaming in my head as it pounded with her non-stop crying.  "Why can't you just SHUT UP!?"  I could feel the anger burning hotter and hotter against this child as I was holding her.  Screaming, sshhhhh, ssshhhh, ssshhhh, screaming, ssshhh, ssshhhh, ssshhh, screaming.  My anger was so bad I was starting to shake...I finally just put my hand over her mouth just to get a break, just for a moment....then I felt her arms hitting my hand in a desperation to get my hand to move so she could breath.  I had kept my hand on her mouth for way too long, and for a moment, just a moment, I didn't want to let go.  She continued to hit my hands, and my brain snapped out of it. I pulled my hand away and she gasped in the much needed air.  I put her gently down in her crib, and walked away sobbing about what I had almost done for just a little quiet.  I didn't pick her up again going forward after that for weeks.  I refused to.  I pushed that all on my wife.  This drove an even bigger wedge between us and the hatred for my daughter continued to grow.

A few weeks after that night, I was working an exhibition event at Century II during a women's show.  I walked by this booth for Scharenberg Chiropractic.  Sign said they could "treat colic".  I scoffed a bit under my breath.  Dr. Scharenberg stopped me and asked why I laughed.  I told him no one could treat that horrible plague.  He told me he could do it.  I said he was a quack and there was no way in hell anyone could do that, I listed off everything we had tried with no success.  He had the audacity to challenge me on it.  The next day was a Sunday.  He told me to be at his office at 6am on a Sunday and he would "prove" to me that he could "fix" my daughter.  He wouldn't even charge me for her treatments.  I said whatever; I'll be there just to spite you.  I had ZERO belief that there was any hope.  I went home and told the wife, and she said I could take her then, but she didn't want any part of it either.  At this point the animosity in our marriage had gotten bad, as I simply didn't help her with the baby since that day.  Big husband fail, but I was too scared I might hurt the baby.

The next day I was at his office, and by goodness, he was there too. We went to the back office after just a bit of paperwork. We sat down with this semi calm (for once) child and he told me that it was going to take some time. He explained he had developed a massage technique over many years and that it would make her really mad as it would cause her some pain, but then she would get the desperately needed relief the child had been screaming for. It was something about an under developed valve. I basically told him to do whatever, because it was just another thing that wouldn't work. He had me feel her gut and it was rock hard. Dr. S. told me babies only cry for certain reasons. They are scared, hungry, or in pain. He said she was in pain from gas being allowed back up in her abdomen from this valve thingy he was going to work on stimulating. Dr. S started his treatment, and boy oh boy, did that baby scream! He worked on her for nearly 45 minutes straight, never raised his voice when talking to her or me, never got angry or impatient, never even doubted. He just kept reassuring us both it would all be okay. The longer he worked on her the angrier I became. I was just about to call it quits, when he looked at me and said "there she goes!" and as I looked down at my daughter, her eyes were super wide, her face super red, holding her breath, and she let out the most incredible fart I had ever heard.  It was at that moment, her face turned back to white and for the most blessed moment in time, she quit crying.  She looked up at him and I as if to say "thank you".  And for the first time since she had been born...not weeks, but months...I saw her smile.  It was as if she were finally in peace as she passed out and went to the first peaceful sleep she had ever had.

My heart broke and I began to weep from both joy and regret.  I never thought that was possible to help her.  I looked at Dr. S and he told me to feel her gut again.  IT WAS SOFT!  He said the pain was released from her.  It would build back up, but he would treat her until her gut was fixed.  That man treated our daughter 2x a day for almost 3 straight weeks.  Even on his days off.  At first, the effects of the treatment only lasted a few hours, and then a few longer hours, and then a whole day, until finally she was relieved.  We had a happy baby to love.  All that time she was just in pain, and I couldn't/didn't know what to do.  I felt like the biggest piece of trash, lousy father in the world. I had hated my child for being in pain. I should have

known....

I wish I could say that all became hunky dory, but the effects of that

colic still linger to this day almost 9 years later. I still get feelings of

anger towards her much quicker than the other 2 children and the

wife and I still have tension around that. Our marriage never quite

recovered from it. However, I do know that I love that girl with my

entire being. I failed her as a father, I almost killed her. I could have

destroyed my family as I let colic ruin our lives. I thank God

constantly for putting Dr. S. in our lives. The miracle of his touch. I

pray that others will be able to continue his technique and bring

peace and relief from suffering to their colic kids and stressed out

family. I truly believe that God works through Dr. Scharenberg's

hands. I have my family. I owe that to Dr. S and his gift of helping

children.

I pray for you reading this. I pray that you can have the patience and

perseverance to learn and execute his technique. It will save your

child and your relationships. You just have to believe. God Bless.

-Anonymous

**So, let's review.**

Colic has had the same criteria since 1954 of a baby crying inconsolably for three hours a day, three days a week, for at least three weeks. There is no pharmaceutical drug recommended for colic, but pediatricians may suggest homeopathic or other soothing remedies to treat the symptoms, not the cause of colic. Sometimes colic symptoms may be a sign of other serious health problems. And, if colic does not resolve itself after a baby is three months old, it is usually diagnosed as acid reflux. Even if babies do outgrow some of the colic symptoms, they generally have digestive problems as children, sometimes even as adults.

The deadliest aspect of colic is the possibility of Shaken Baby Syndrome. Although parents and caregivers don't intend to hurt their babies, a combination of factors, including stress and fatigue, causes 1,400 babies a year to die from Shaken Baby Syndrome. In response to this crisis, "Period of PURPLE crying" was created to encourage and give coping strategies to parents and caregivers; however, it does not address the cause of colic.

**A new definition and approach for colic**

There is something wrong with the current colic diagnosis, which has been used for years, as it has yet to describe or treat the major cause of colic. How would I redefine the definition of colic and what is the major cause of colic? Colic comes from the word "colon" and generally is the result of a weak ileocecal valve between the small and large intestines. If the valve is too weak and does not close properly, digestion repeats itself in the small intestine. Gas builds up creating sharp pain. Babies can begin to exhibit symptoms as early as just a few days old. Many babies may exhibit symptoms of colic without the parents realizing the cause of the problem. Most people believe that the only sign of colic is when a baby cries excessively; however, some babies suffering from colic may only grunt or have trouble sleeping. In order to help your baby, first you need to determine if your baby's crying is being caused by colic.

I have spent forty years taking care of babies with colic. Through this I have learned a true, gentle way of treating and relieving a baby's discomfort without spinal manipulation. I have also learned patience, as the treatment works only if it is consistently done. I stay with the treatment of every patient until the parents confirm complete satisfaction. When the treatment is done correctly, babies will find relief from colic symptoms in about two weeks.

I love babies and my passion is to relieve them of this deadly, awful, painful condition. It is that passion which has led me to share this book with you. I encourage you to read it all the way through and share with other families who have an infant suffering from colic. If your child has one or many of the symptoms listed above, he or she may be suffering from colic. In my practice, I have seen thousands of babies suffering in varying degrees with the symptoms above. The one thing they have all had in common is a parent or caregiver who felt something wasn't right and sought out my treatment. If you feel your baby is in pain, trust your gut. Reading this book is the first step to getting help for your baby.

## Checklist of colic symptoms

Think your baby may have colic? If you can say, "yes" to any of the listed symptoms, your baby may be part of the 40% of babies who suffer from colic.[1]

- Inability to stay latched on to the breast or bottle
- Pain when passing flatulence and stool (liquid or formed)
- Scratching of the face, ears, head, and pulling his or her hair
- Inability to lie flat on back without crying
- Not wanting to take a pacifier
- Vomiting, either projectile or just spitting up usually frequently (Usually diagnosed as acid reflux or silent reflux)
- Sleeping at odd hours, usually described as having days and nights mixed up
- Crying sounds mostly high pitch and variable with high and lows

- Always wanting to have motion such as swings or bouncing
- Always wanting to be held in an upright position
- When being held, trying to crawl up over the adult's shoulder
- Always wanting to be taken for a ride, calming down with motion and crying when the vehicle stops
- Kicking the legs most frequently the left leg (This is an attempt to help move the descending colon)
- Usually diagnosed as lactose intolerant
- Symptoms starts at variety of times from birth to 6 weeks

| Checklist of colic symptoms (continued) ||
|---|---|
| <ul><li>Grunting</li><li>Fussing</li><li>Crying</li><li>Kicking of the legs</li><li>Flaring of the arms</li><li>Arching of the back</li><li>Distention of the abdomen</li><li>Inability to stay latched on to the breast or the bottle</li><li>Decreased bowel motion</li></ul> | <ul><li>Developing umbilical hernia (an "outie" bellybutton)</li><li>Continually wanting to suck</li><li>Rooting and sucking</li><li>Decreased bowel motion</li><li>Negative upper and lower GI studies</li></ul> |
| <ul><li>Symptoms can last for months and years and after 1 year is usually diagnosed as something other than colic such as colitis, irritable bowel, indigestion, heart burn, gastritis, Crohn's, chronic constipation, chronic diarrhea.</li><li>Always stiff and rigid body with clenched hands and contracted arms and legs</li></ul> | <ul><li>Decreased weight gain: underfed because of pain</li><li>Increased weight gain: overfed because of pain</li><li>Eventually hemorrhoids or rectal fissures (tear in the lining of the lower rectum)</li><li>Crying with eyes closed</li><li>Not sleeping except for short periods</li></ul> |

## Chapter 2: Is Acid Reflux Colic?

### *Common misdiagnoses for colic*

### My story

I didn't know how to fix the crying babies when I first started my practice. But the thing was, no one else knew how to fix them either. There was no one to help these crying babies. I had been trained in college to treat adults for various digestive issues such as leaky gut, irritable bowel, etc. The more I watched the babies come in with a lot of bloating and screaming, I realized there had to be a digestive connection. I started hitting the books, reading all the published information about the gastrointestinal tract. Then, I started to do clinical hours with the babies. I spent hundreds of hours with babies, not looking to remedy colic, but looking for something that would help. As I talked with my patients' parents on why they decided to seek my help, a common thread was that they had initially turned to their pediatrician for help. After three months of crying, medical authorities started looking for other reasons as to why the baby was crying. Many parents shared a story like this--perhaps you can understand the frustration:

Three months have passed. Allison's baby is still crying, especially in the evening. He spits up after every meal, and the spit up is not little and cute. It is projectile. It covers everything! Allison is up to her ears in laundry, and her husband accidently comments that she always smells like sour milk, then realizing his mistake, quickly offers to do some laundry. But, both Allison and her husband think the worst part of the situation is their little baby. Face red, eyes squinting. When will he get some relief? Allison mentions her concerns again to her pediatrician. He suggests the possibility of acid reflux and offers giving her baby tests to confirm. Fear seizes her heart as questions flood her head. What could this mean for her baby?

If your baby was given a diagnosis like the one above, some of the questions you might have asked are the following: What is acid reflux? Why are so many people bothered by it? Is it serious? Why is it so common? What causes it? What are the symptoms? What is the treatment? Can it be cured? How is it diagnosed? Does it run in families? Can it be prevented?

As with colic, there is much confusion over gastroesophageal reflux disease, also known as GERD. In my experience, only a small percentage of the babies who are diagnosed with GERD actually have the disease; most infants are dealing with a weak ileocecal valve between the small and large intestines, which creates unbearable symptoms similar to that of acid reflux. These babies are suffering from colic, misdiagnosed as GERD.

## GERD

But first, just what is GERD? GERD, also known as gastroesophageal reflux, is chronic or severe acid reflux. Acid reflux is a regurgitation or fluid coming back up the esophagus from the stomach, whether it be milk, saliva, or even formed food particles. Acid that is formed in the stomach may also come back up with belching or vomiting, either by itself or mixed with other food substances. Acid, of course, causes an irritation to the stomach and esophagus, which can cause swelling, which in time causes pain. Until it becomes painful, it doesn't usually get our attention. So this consistent acid reflux, usually when it is causing pain, is called GERD.

When we have health problems, we figure out what is hurting and maybe how we can reduce the swelling and pain, but what is usually not understood is the cause of the problem. The big question is why does acid come back up?

If you go online and look for the etiology, the cause of most diseases, you will find that for a majority of diseases, the causes are simply unknown. For example:

1. What is asthma and what causes it?

2. What is fibromyalgia and what is causing it?

3. What is cancer and what is causing it?

4. What is a stomach ulcer (gastritis) and what is causing it?

The answer is frequently, "We just don't know."

**Acid reflux and babies**

So let's dive into acid reflux and how it relates to babies. Why is acid reflux a problem? It's because of the acid. When a baby vomits, it is usually milk, which dilutes stomach acid coming up the esophagus and doesn't cause any damage. If there is a large amount of acid that is not diluted, it can cause burning. If the burning continues over an extended period of time, this can cause damage to the cells, and when the baby becomes an adult, this continued damage to the cells could eventually cause cancer.

The question still remains: why does the acid want to keep

coming back up the esophagus? Another question sometimes

forgotten is what is causing the reflux?

Like mentioned above, acid reflux graduates to GERD when

acid (or regurgitation) in the reflux causes irritation or injury to the

esophagus. Most authorities believe this occurs only in a small

percentage of infants who spit up frequently or spit up in large

amounts. Symptoms most often seen are:

1. Refusing to eat

2. Frequent crying

3. Arching the neck and back indicating severe pain (this is a

major symptom of colic)

4. Projectile vomiting

5. Choking

6. Coughing

7. Unable to gain normal weight

There are medical diagnostic tests to give more information on

how severe the problem is or how much damage has already occurred

such as barium swallow or PH probe. Normal medical treatment

given, depending on the severity of the reflux, is Zantac, Prilosec,

Tagamet, etc. Most studies demonstrate that reflux does not usually cause pain in infants and reducing stomach acid does not decrease irritability. If the baby continues to have the above symptoms, then more in depth testing can be done such as blood and urine tests, x-ray studies of the digestive tract, and possibly a test called endoscopy which will allow the physician to view the lining of the esophagus. Studies indicate that at least 80% of the babies with these symptoms will partially or completely improve without any medical intervention.[1]

**When acid reflux is actually colic**

Does position of an individual make a difference in acid reflux? With adults, as well as with children and babies, a recumbent position will aggravate the acid reflux. Adults with acid reflux report that their most severe episodes will occur when they are lying on their back. The more severe incidents seem to occur at night when they are asleep. They wake up out of a sound sleep, start coughing violently, and notice liquid coming up the esophagus. Some of the reflux may get into the bronchial tubes and lungs. This burns and hurts. Adults may immediately stand up and get a drink of water to help reduce the burning of the throat. Babies, in contrast, will usually spit up or projectile vomit, and then without coughing, go immediately back to drinking without any problems.

Spitting up is one of the most common symptoms of colic. What usually happens is parents will take their baby to the pediatrician to find out why their baby is spitting up. The pediatrician will exam the baby and in most cases will not find any obvious reason. No fever, no ear infections, heart and lung sounds are clear, no sinus infections, and no skin rash. The baby appears to be healthy, but the baby may have a distended abdomen and other symptoms common to colic. The doctor will send them home reassuring them that the baby is healthy and may tell the parents that spitting up to some degree is normal. He will encourage them to burp the baby more often and try not to overfeed.

The parents will take the child home, but the problem continues. The parents are very worried about their baby and will continue to take the baby back to the pediatrician. Since there are no medications other than gas drops, simethicone drops, or other homeopathic remedies, the doctor might suggest one of these remedies and send them home reassuring them that the colic will go away in an average of three months or less. The parents may then return to the pediatrician again in tears and more forcibly push the doctor to find out what is wrong with their baby.

The parents are scared, sleep deprived, and losing faith in their doctor because their baby isn't getting better. The parents search the web and ask others for advice. Many times they will seek the advice of another pediatrician, frantically hoping to find a way to get their baby well. The doctor might make a diagnosis of acid reflux and prescribe Zantac, Prilosec, Tagamet, or some other antacid.

The medicine may help reduce the symptoms for a short time, but in two or three days the symptoms seem to get worse again. The acid reflux medicine does not stop the spitting up or the vomiting. Instead, it is supposed to decrease the drainage to the esophagus and stomach, hoping to prevent more serious problems in the future. My experience with antacid medications is that they will not improve or change colic symptoms.

How long are babies kept on this medication? If the results do not indicate any improvement in three or four weeks, then pediatricians usually recommend stopping. At this time the pediatrician may recommend a referral to a pediatric gastroenterologist for further examination and tests. The frustrating diagnosis may be the following: the baby is healthy. Take the baby home, and in three months, the colic or "acid reflux" will go away.

**Esophageal Hiatal Hernias**

Once in a while, acid reflux is the correct diagnosis, which is generally caused by an esophageal hiatal hernia. If this is the finding, then appropriate medications or surgery will be recommended; however, this does not occur frequently. When it does happen, parents will be sent home with instructions on conservative care until the baby outgrows the symptoms. Colic and acid reflux are both very frustrating conditions for everyone: the baby, the parents, and the doctors.

What we have found with acid reflux or esophageal hiatal hernias is that pressure from the lower abdomen is pushing part of the stomach and/or intestines up into the hiatus, or hole, in the diaphragm between the heart and lungs, and the stomach and intestines. This is, many times, the result of the pressure in the intestines from the colic, which is caused by the leakage of the ileocecal valve. This leakage causes digested material from the large intestine to be re-digested, causing bloating and distention of the large and small intestine. This causes the colic symptoms not other things like milk or a lactose intolerant problem.

This pressure pushing the stomach and/or intestine up into the hiatus that the esophagus comes through, creates a squeezing or constriction of the lower end of the esophagus. The esophagus is a muscle contracting tube, which if squeezed or narrowed can cause severe substernal pain. Many times in an adult this is mistaken for a heart attack.

The other symptom that is experienced is a feeling in the throat that the food and sometimes just normal saliva won't go down and can't be swallowed. This gives a choking feeling and causes a gagging sound in the throat. What a baby will do is arch his back, tilt his head back (usually to the right), and make gagging or choking sounds. This is what acid reflux looks and sounds like. This is also true in an adult; however, the adult will usually bend forward and grab their chest at the substernal location (at the end of the sternum or chest) and complain of severe chest pain and the inability to swallow.

This happens in adults when they drink, take pills, or bend over too much, which can cause the stomach or intestine to push up into the esophageal hiatus and cause this compression to the end of the esophagus. Medical treatment of anti-acid therapy, such as Zantac, is of little use at this point. The cause of acid reflux is not the absence of Zantac; it is the pressure against the esophagus causing the problems and pain.

The treatment we have found that is most effective most of the time is to use a pressure technique to remove the stomach and/or intestine from the hiatus in the diaphragm. I have used this technique most of my career, and it is effective most of the time. When this technique works in babies, the pain and spitting up symptoms go away. This technique is very effective in adults as well.

There are many pediatricians who disagree with these results; however, if you had pain in your big toe because someone was standing on it, what would make more sense? Making the person get off your big toe or taking medication to attempt to relieve the pain? In my opinion and experience, it seems more effective to physically remove the pressure against the esophagus with a physical or mechanical treatment. More discussion of this technique will be given in training videos, which complement this book.

## Other causes of crying

One thing that makes colic so frustrating is that crying can be the first complaint of any disease in infants. How can you tell the difference between colic and something more serious? The statistics may be in your baby's favor. After reviewing over 30 years of literature dealing with colic, researchers say that less than 5% of colic cases have to do with organic disease, which is a disease caused by a physical change in the structure of an organ or body part. That 5% includes intolerance to cow's milk, fructose intolerance, fluoxetine hydrochloride (an antidepressant better known as Prozac that can transfer to mom's milk), migraines, reflux esophagitis (which is associated with GERD), infant abuse, lactose intolerance, glaucoma, central nervous system abnormalities, and urinary tract infection.[2]

An intolerance to mother's milk as a result of the mother's diet or an intolerance to prepared formula seems to be a frequent diagnosis for crying babies with digestive distress, explained as allergies or lactose intolerance. Mothers are told to stop dairy and see if the baby improves. If that doesn't help, parents may be asked to switch to goat's milk instead of mother's milk. Of all the babies I have treated in forty years, only a very small number of mothers and babies were adversely affected by dairy in their diet. This is another common misdiagnosis.

Beyond GERD, organic diseases and allergies, there are many other illnesses that could be causing a baby distress. The illness may also be coupled with colic. Although this is not an exhaustive list, here are some of the illnesses that can affect babies: sinus infection, ear infection, bronchial infection, pneumonia (or other respiratory problem), teething, chronic constipation, chronic diarrhea which leads to dehydration, or injury from the birthing process. Watching your baby closely and giving your pediatrician a list of symptoms will help diagnose infections. Injuries from the birthing process are also a possible source of pain and could include broken clavicles, arms, legs, or possibly ribs. Sometimes cervical spine injuries also happen. These aren't always diagnosed after the baby is born. Another spinal condition is Torticollis, which is when a baby's head pulls to one side, which could be the result of an injury before or during birth. Other reasons for Torticollis include unequal head position in car seats or while sleeping, or from extreme temperature changes (from heat to cold too quickly). These illnesses, although serious, are not very common.

Can you treat a baby who has colic coupled with another illness? Absolutely. In some cases, treating the colic may accelerate the healing of the other disease or may eliminate the illness all together. As mentioned earlier, the key here is to be a detective who closely observes your baby. Keep track of symptoms and behaviors. If you suspect GERD or any of the illnesses or physical injuries mentioned in this chapter, keep speaking with your pediatrician. Get as much information as you can to make an informed decision. For most babies, my colic treatment works with reduced symptoms within two weeks; however, if a baby isn't responding as expected, then the baby may be suffering from something else.

My colic treatment is not a spinal manipulation or adjustment. The treatment strengthens the ileocecal valve, the valve between the small and large intestines. Like developing any muscle, the strengthening takes time and patience. In my office, the treatment usually lasts two weeks, and I see the baby every day. But, when a baby has another ailment, the treatment may take longer. This is especially true for failure to thrive babies.

**Failure to thrive babies**

The term "failure to thrive" may be given by a pediatrician and refers to the "failure" to meet growth milestones in weight and height. It could point to an underlying health issue, but like the term "colic," it is more of a description than diagnosis of a specific problem. The biggest concern for failure to thrive babies is that they are undernourished.

These babies react and have colic just like many other babies; however, they don't improve as quickly when treated and cannot eat well. Eating seems to hurt them, and they often show signs that the milk is hard to swallow. The pain seems to be more in the stomach (under the left rib cage) than in the lower abdomen. They spit up frequently and their cry sounds so painful. Their appearance is different; they are usually small, don't gain weight, become more dehydrated, and their faces may look like little old men.

When I treat these babies, they feel relief from the colic treatment, but they usually will not reach the same full health like other babies. They usually continue to cry because they are not getting enough nutrition as a result of being unable to keep milk down. Many of these babies must use NG tubes or G tubes in order to receive a sufficient amount of nutrients for survival. Working with your pediatrician closely will ensure your baby receives the nutrition he or she needs to thrive.

**So, let's review.**

GERD is chronic acid reflux. Babies may be given this diagnosis when colic symptoms do not subside. The treatment for GERD includes a prescription of Zantac, Prilosec, Tagamet, or some other antacid. Although these medicines do not stop the spit up or projectile vomit symptoms, the medicines neutralize the acid, avoiding further damage to the esophagus or stomach. Many times this diagnosis is given even though the baby only has colic.

When acid reflux is the correct diagnosis, it is usually because of an esophageal hiatal hernia. The pressure from the lower abdomen is pushing part of the stomach and or intestines up in the hiatus (hole) in the diaphragm between the the heart and lungs, and the stomach and intestines. Although in infants most acid reflux resolves itself, the best treatment is to remove the stomach or intestine from the hole in the diaphragm. This is done through a pressure technique, and when effective, the pain and spitting up symptoms go away.

Another diagnosis often given for colicky babies is a food allergy or intolerance. Breastfeeding mothers are usually told to avoid dairy. Or, a formula-fed baby might be given goat's milk. This is also usually a misdiagnosis.

There are many other common illnesses that could cause distress to a baby including injury during birth. These may be the main causes of distress for a baby, or the illness could be coupled with colic.

Parents today need to be detectives. Recording symptoms and finding a pediatrician who listens to all concerns is imperative. The more a parent can address the reason a baby is uncomfortable or in pain, the more he or she can do something about it. What I have learned after many years of practice is that when it comes to health issues, fear plays a major role.

Fear comes from ignorance of the facts. It is impossible to know everything about everything, so we are all ignorant about many things. Asking lots of questions and looking for answers is one way parents can help their children. I believe one of the major reasons humans tend to be so uninformed about health issues is because generally people look at the human body and believe it is too complicated to learn about.

For the most part, we have been educated about how to relieve symptoms, but we don't know what the symptoms are telling us about our bodies. For example, pain. We all know what it feels like and our major concern is how to get rid of it, not what is causing it and what is actually hurting. What people don't realize is what typically causes pain is swelling. In general, the amount of pain you experience is directly related to how much swelling is present.

What is not always understood is that most pain pills are called *anti* meaning "against" and *inflammatory* meaning "swelling." What health care professionals know is that when you reduce the swelling, you will reduce the pain. The medicine may reduce the swelling for a while, but if the root cause of the swelling is not taken care of, the swelling will return.

Once you determine the cause (or causes) of why your baby is crying, choose a treatment that will address the problem, not just the symptoms. Your baby will thank you.

# Testimonial

Hudson is our second child to receive colic treatment from Dr. Scharenberg. I was referred to him by a co-worker when I started having suspicions that my daughter really didn't have acid reflux as diagnosed by her pediatrician. From two weeks on she had to be constantly held and was incredibly fussy during the early evening hours. We did a lot of walking and bouncing!

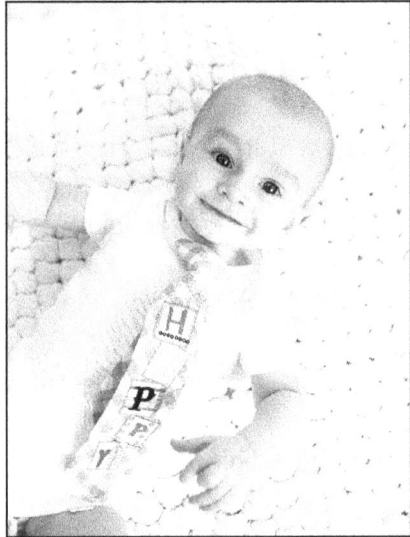

Tension was very high in our house! We brought Adeline to his office when she was 5 weeks old and noticed a drastic difference in her after just two treatments. I was breastfeeding, so I immediately changed my diet and followed Doc's plan. She had more treatments than average even though I was very strict with the diet, but the last few weeks of treatment were just getting from 75% to 100% better. I had to continue to avoid certain foods such as chocolate and caffeine for a few more months, but eventually could eat whatever I wanted.

Because of our experience with Adeline, we recognized the colic symptoms in Hudson right away.  He was initially very gassy and restless and did not want to sleep on his back, so we brought him to Doc when he was a week old and began treatments right away.  Fortunately, he never got to the painful crying and loss of sleep stage!  Because we started so early, things moved much more quickly and he was 'cured' in about 2 weeks.  I was also breastfeeding him, but this time I started adjusting my diet from the time he was born as a preventative measure.  Doing this also helped me determine which foods bothered him more than others, and I continued to avoid those until he was a little older.

With both of our babies, there was an immediate improvement; however, we did experience a regression during treatment for a few days.  That was then followed by more improvement.  The temporary modification to my diet was completely worth it too.  We are so grateful for Doc's colic treatment, which gave us happy babies and made us happy parents!

Mom: Heather Hatcher

# Chapter 3: Is there Colic Medicine I Can Give My Baby?

## *Homeopathic medicine and other chemical "remedies" explained*

### My story

Common sense. That's what I kept coming back to as I studied what could help colicky babies. When I was a little boy, my father heard that swabbing infected tonsils with kerosene would get rid of a sore throat. This was an old wives' tale that could have done incredible harm to me. Likewise, there are many myths associated with how to treat colicky babies. For example, another old wives' tale of giving whiskey to a colicky baby does not make sense and would be very harmful.

The historic definition of colic, a diagnosis for a crying baby, does not answer the question of why the baby cries. So, developing a medicine to correct the crying is difficult. Over the years many people have stated that they have found various solutions for colic based on their theories of what causes colic; however, the overall opinion is that these medicines are ineffective and unpredictable. This is true for both more traditional medicine and homeopathic remedies. The information given in this chapter is meant to educate, not to prescribe or diagnose. I am not recommending any of these techniques because I have seen many parents who have tried them with little results. However, many parents have questions about the various methods below. This chapter was written to help explain them.

**Herbs and Homeopathy**

Herbs and other homeopathic remedies were some of human's first treatments for everyday ailments like headaches and sore muscles. With the modernization of medicine, these treatments have taken a backseat to pharmaceutical drugs, and today we are more likely to reach for an aspirin than peppermint (*menta piperita*) for a headache. However, because there is no pharmaceutical drug for colic, many have looked to nature and medicine's past for relief.

Herbs, unlike chemical medicine that treats symptoms, aim to treat the cause of the problem. In simplistic terms, herbs are believed to encourage the body to heal itself by promoting different bodily functions through nutrients. Many herbs given to adults are not safe for infants. So, it is with extreme caution that these ingredients are given to infants, and, in my experience, not with much success.

Herbs are used in the form of capsules, powders, teas, or

glycerin extracts.[1] They may be made from a plant's leaves, roots, stems, or flowers.[2] A traditional remedy for colic is fennel (*Foeniculum vulgare*) tea, given to breastfeeding mothers. There are some studies which show tea with fennel may help babies by relieving gas and relaxing the gastrointestinal tract.[3] Other herbs which may be used in remedies include slippery elm (*Ulmus fulva*), chamomile (*Matricaria recutita*), lemon balm (*Melissa officinalis*), linden (*Tilia cordata*), catnip (*Nepeta cataria*), peppermint (*Mentha piperita*), and dill (*Anethum graveolens*). They are used for their calming and soothing effects on a baby's digestive system.

A common commercial product is homeopathic gripe water, which has been used for over a hundred years. Homeopathy is a term given to medicine acknowledged by the FDA that has a more natural and nontoxic content. Gripe water contains ginger, caraway, fennel, peppermint, lemon balm, chamomile, and blackthorn, among other ingredients (depending on the brand). These ingredients are added for their gas relief or digestive aid. The original gripe water recipe included alcohol, which old wives' tales recommended. However, studies prove that alcohol is not effective.[4] The FDA ensures that none of the brands sold in the U.S. include alcohol, which should not be given to babies.

In my experience, the use of herbs, gripe water, or other homeopathic remedies may temporarily help a baby, but the colic symptoms return. Most parents who I work with have tried and given up on gripe water, gas drops, or other homeopathic treatments. The reason? The relief doesn't seem to last, and, although the side effects are usually harmless, one of my patient's parents was alarmed after giving her baby gripe water for several consecutive days. Black deposits started to show up in her infant's diaper. Although there were no other side effects, she immediately stopped the treatment and started my colic treatment instead.

**Drug Therapies**

Simethicone (Mylicon) is an over-the-counter gas remedy that is sometimes recommended for colic. It is said "to relieve symptoms of extra gas caused by air swallowing or certain foods/infant formulas. [It] helps break up gas bubbles in the gut."[5] There are generally no side effects with this medicine; however, although rare, allergic reactions can occur. What I have found is that the baby might find temporary relief, but the symptoms return, similar to homeopathic remedies.

Although not a drug, a popular recommendation from pediatricians is to give the baby 7up or seltzer water. The idea is that the carbonation would help move any air or gas and bring more comfort to the baby. What I would caution about this approach is how this might elevate the baby's blood sugar if given regularly.

Carbonated water seems to cause an increase in bloating, not a decrease. Therefore, if breastfeeding, I would recommend eliminating all carbonated drinks from the mom's diet until the baby has been treated and the colic eliminated.

## Probiotics

There has been a lot of excitement about the discovery of how gut flora affects the body and the use of probiotics. Gut flora (also known as gut microbiota) is a population of microorganisms that reside in the intestines. There are tens of trillions of microorganisms in every person, with one-third of the gut flora being common to most people and the remaining two-thirds unique to the individual. Think of it as your individualized fingerprint, from your gut.

Gut flora helps the body digest certain foods, produce vitamins, maintain the wholeness of the intestinal mucosa, and play a role in protecting the immune system.[6] The gut flora is shaped by what we come in contact with after birth. Gut flora continues to change throughout our lives and reflects our diets and environments. It can adapt to change, but sometimes dysbiosis, a loss of balance in gut flora, can occur. This loss of balance is linked to illnesses such as functional bowel disorder, inflammatory bowel disease, allergies, obesity, and diabetes.

This is where probiotics and prebiotics come into play. The difference between the two is found in living microbes. Probiotics, found in several fermented foods like yogurt, contain living microbes. Prebiotics do not. Prebiotics contain non-digestible food particles that promote the growth of friendly microbes already in the gut flora[7] and are "food" for beneficial bacteria.[6] Or, in simplistic terms, they are the offense, while probiotics are the defense. Probiotics are thought to work in different ways, including preventing bad bacteria growth, blocking bad bacteria, and enhancing the immune system.[7]

There are several studies that have looked at how

microorganisms relating to the intestines differ in colicky babies.[8,9] So, it is with that in mind that professionals have turned to probiotics, specifically lactobacillus reuteri. In a randomized, double-blind, placebo-controlled trial, infants given the probiotic cried 50% less.[10] Likewise, another study comparing probiotics and simethicone found infants given lactobacillus reuteri improved faster than their peers given simethicone.[11] These studies are not reporting complete improvement, though. It is still not understood how exactly probiotics treat colic or how the gut flora influences other parts of overall health. There is still more research and discovery to be had in this area.

If a baby I am treating is on probiotics, I ask that the parents discontinue until the treatment is done. Because my method is a mechanical one, instead of chemical, I like to have the baby off anything that may contribute to the weakening of the valve. My job is to fix the baby so it doesn't need anything for their digestive distress, including medicine or another chemical form.

## Alternative Health Services

Although alternative health services are usually not ingested like the chemical treatments mentioned above, I get a lot of questions regarding the science and results of different types of alternative health services. Let me explain a little about what sets them apart and why I think people may be unsure of using their services.

Alternative health services are the name given to health practices that are not standard medical practices. They are sometimes labeled as "preventative" or "therapeutic." Reflexology, acupuncture, acupressure, and chiropractic care are types of alternative health services.

Within each type of alternative health service are many differing philosophies and techniques. That's why going to one chiropractor may be a different experience than going to another. As a chiropractor, I am open to whatever treatments I believe will benefit my patients, even the smallest patients. I have studied acupuncture and acupressure. And, there are many times babies need adjustments after birth. The birthing process can be difficult for babies, and the realigning of the spine through manual adjustment may make a big difference.

But most people are apprehensive about allowing their baby to be "adjusted, poked, or prodded," as one mom told me. If a parent has never been treated by an alternative health professional themselves, he or she will hesitate to treat their baby. According to a survey, 37% of the U.S. population have tried chiropractic care, but only 15% see their chiropractic doctor yearly.[12] It is the 85% of the American population whom do not regularly see chiropractors that I have written this book for.

Even though I am a chiropractor, my colic treatment is not an adjustment or spinal manipulation. It is a technique that strengthens the ileocecal valve. Through strengthening the valve, symptoms are reduced until there is a reduction of symptoms and parents are satisfied with the progress. The colic symptoms are relieved. While other treatments need to be performed by professionals, my treatment is easy to learn and can be done from the comfort of the baby's home.

> If you do seek out reflexology, acupuncture, acupressure, or chiropractic care services, do your research. Select a reputable practitioner who has experience with infants.

**So, let's review.**

There are several claims on how to calm colicky babies from medicines to herbs. Studies show that some techniques are more effective than others, but they all only claim to reduce colic symptoms, not eliminate colic. Herbs, probiotics, and over-the-counter medicines are all chemical approaches to treating colic. They rely on the body reacting positively to the substance introduced (whether dermally or internally).

A more physical approach would be using reflexology, acupuncture, acupressure, or chiropractic care. These types of health care are called alternative health care. Many are unsure about these types of services and are apprehensive about letting their little infants receive care. That is why I reassure parents that there is a gentle, effective way to treat colic.

My colic treatment is a physical approach, but it is not a spinal manipulation or adjustment. It is a gentle technique that strengthens the ileocecal valve over time. It not only reduces colic symptoms, but it goes beyond what other strategies boast and relieves the colic.

## <u>Testimonial</u>

From what I have heard before I had

Madison, colic was something many parents

feared. Madison would cry and cry,

sometimes screaming cries, and nothing that

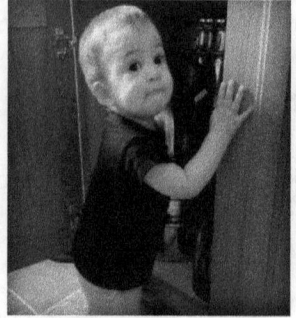

mommy or daddy did would help this. Eventually I think she was so

worn out from crying that she would fall asleep. My baby was only 2

months old at the time, and I knew I needed help. Madison's

pediatrician told me to buy gas drops and to just keep rocking her and

trying to soothe her. She basically told me that she would eventually

grow out of it and for now to just keep doing what I was doing. Both

Madison and I were getting very little sleep, and I was feeling

hopeless.

One day I asked my Facebook friends for advice on colic, and

my uncle replied that he took my cousins to Dr. Scharenberg. I called

the Doc's office immediately and got set up for an evaluation that

next day.

My initial thoughts of taking my daughter to a chiropractor

were a little skeptical; however, I was so exhausted that I was more than ready to try something different. After the initial visit, my Madison took a 4-hour nap! Before that day she was sleeping 30 minutes for naps.

Because I was breastfeeding, I had to follow the diet, which was difficult, but I kept in mind that it was only for 2 weeks. I did veer from the diet a couple of times with caffeine. One night, I had to go to the Doc's house for a treatment because Madison had been crying all day long. I was in tears but after the treatment she went home and slept all night.

There was a point during the treatment when I felt like Madison's improvements started regressing. I started feeling skeptical again. However, after the next couple of treatment days, Madison started improving again.

I took Madison to the Doc for a total of about 12 treatments, but I think the last few treatments were more for me to feel sure that Madison's colic was gone. The colic was in fact gone and Madison has been so happy ever since. I feel so blessed that the Doc was there to help us.      Mom: Dana Thomas

# Chapter 4: How Do I Soothe My Baby?

## *Soothing techniques explained*

**My Story**

By the time I see parents, many are so frustrated because they have been given so much conflicting advice on how to calm their baby. Everything that they've tried hasn't worked because their colicky infant is in pain. As we go through the treatment, the babies have less pain, and the parents are better able to comfort them. Having a collection of soothing strategies in your pocket and understanding why they are soothing is beneficial. It can help you be more confident as a caregiver, especially as you find what works best for your baby. Like mentioned in the previous chapter, it is also important to use common sense when deciding how to soothe your baby.

Today's champion for soothing techniques is pediatrician Dr. Harvey Karp. His approach to alleviating colic symptoms has to do with strategies on how to comfort the baby. Many of these strategies have been handed down for generations and are natural to parents. Let's take a look at Dr. Karp's popular 5 S's, along with other soothing techniques, and some older home remedies, which your grandmother might have used.

## Dr. Karp's 5 S's[7]

Dr. Karp's *The Happiest Baby on the Block* discusses the 5 S's, or 5 main soothing techniques, for easing baby's crying. He also discusses colic in his book, but he has never claimed to eliminate the condition of colic. Dr. Karp's theory on the source behind colic goes back to evolution. He feels that babies were once born at 12 months gestation, but because of evolution, are now born at 9 months. This missing trimester creates a premature digestive system. His logic follows that since colic is only supposed to last up to 3 months, then if a baby was born at 12 months, these problems associated with colic would no longer exist. I applaud Dr. Karp's efforts for giving caregivers strategies to soothe their babies. In my experience, these soothing techniques are helpful in periodically calming the crying; however, they do not seem to be effective in curing colic in the long term (especially if your baby's colic lasts longer than 3 months).

## Swaddling

The idea of swaddling (and all of Dr. Karp's 5 S's) is that it mimics the environment that the baby felt in the womb. It is true that when babies are born they usually have startle reflexes for the first few weeks of their life (also known as moro reflexes). As babies get to know their environment, they might startle from a sudden move or sound or feeling. The startle reflex lasts only a second and might include the baby flinging his arms and legs. As newborns sleep 16 to 22 hours a day, this startle can wake them up. Swaddling keeps their arms and legs confined so that the startle reflex is less disruptive to them.[1]

My experience with swaddling is that if the colic pain is severe and the abdomen is large and tight, many times swaddling will make it worse. If you were bloated and someone tied your arms and legs down, would you like it? You would want to relieve the pressure on your abdomen, not make it tighter. You also wouldn't want your arms and legs tied; you would want to move as much as you could. That's why babies kick and flail their arms; it gives them a little relief. Occasionally, swaddling may calm a baby down; however, more times than not, it could make the pain worse. If you want to swaddle your baby, don't secure the blanket too tight. This is also true to prevent hip dysplasia.[2]

On another note, colicky babies have more pain when laying on their backs, so if you swaddle your baby and then put her on her back, you will most likely be causing more pain. This is tough, because for safe sleep, the American Academy of Pediatricians recommends that infants be placed on their backs.[3] What's a caregiver to do?

**Side or stomach**

This is referencing holding the baby on his side or stomach. Whenever you change the baby's position, it will cause the air in the stomach and intestines to move and then will release some distended pressure on the stomach. If you had an excessive amount of gas in the stomach or in the intestines, what would you do? You would probably roll over to your side and bring your knees up to your chest. This would change some of the pressure on the intestines. You would get some relief; however, my guess is that you wouldn't stay in that position very long. Moving around will probably relieve some pain, but it won't fix the problem. This is another reason why swaddling a baby tight could cause more pain because it keeps them from moving, which can help move the gas around.

Being on the stomach puts pressure on the abdomen, which could definitely increase the pain; however, it can also have the opposite effect by helping move the feces farther through the intestine and relieve some pressure. I have discussed this with hundreds of parents and have found that babies many times will actually get relief by lying down on their stomachs. As for Sudden Infant Death Syndrome (SIDS), I have not found any explanations as to why experts think stomach sleeping causes SIDS except that it easier for babies to press their face into the mattress. The fact is that there are a lot of theories surrounding SIDS but no definite proof of what causes it. The American Pediatrics Association reports that since 1992 when they recommended that babies sleep on their back, there has been a dramatic decline of SIDS; however, "sleep-related deaths from other causes, including suffocation, entrapment and asphyxia, have increased."[3]

My question is this: If you had a baby who was prone to projectile vomiting and was lying on his back, possibly swaddled, he probably wouldn't be able to move. So if he vomited, what would he do? He couldn't move, he couldn't turn his head to the side, he couldn't roll over. So what would be the most likely thing to happen? After he vomits, he would then take a deep breath and try to cry. The milk would most likely come right back in his face. He would then take another deep breath, which could aspirate the milk right into his lungs. This would not be good.

If he was on his side or stomach and not swaddled, what would he do? Most likely he would turn his head and the milk would run down, allowing him to breathe. The chances of aspirating milk would be far less. What I am saying is that I believe this concept needs a lot more research so parents can make the best decisions for their babies.

### Shushing

Shushing is a normal response by parents to distract babies in hopes that they will stop crying. Dr. Karp explains shushing as being a reassurance to babies because it reminds them of the womb. Is the baby comforted because the sound reminds him of the sound of blood flow when he was in utero? Perhaps. It definitely distracts the baby some, and if the pain is not severe, it seems to help; however, if the gas pressure is more excessive and the pain is more severe, then no sound seems to help. Will shushing hurt the baby? No. So my advice is, if it does no harm, then go ahead. Anything you can do to help your baby stop crying is worth a try.

Another approach parents use is the sound of white noise from a vacuum or sound machine. Again, if it does no harm, then go for it. However, be cautious as to the volume and proximity to your baby's ears. A 2014 study looked at the decibel levels of several popular infant sound machines and found that many were capable of producing volume levels capable of causing harm.[4] Although the study did not look at the effects the high volume had on babies, the study's overall message was that parents should exercise caution when using machines to produce ambient noise. Be considerate of the volume and proximity to your baby's ears. And, if you are using an infant sound machine, be sure to follow the manufacturer's instructions.

**Swinging**

Car rides, stroller walks, and swings all mimic the fluid movement that baby felt inside the womb, rocking in the amniotic fluid. The biggest reason I believe swinging helps is because it changes the amount of gas pressure on certain spots of the stomach and intestines, like positioning the baby on her side or stomach. It helps relieve the pain because the gas has the opportunity to move.

It's like if you drove your car into a lake (an example, not a suggestion). All the air would go to the top of the car. It would be trapped in the roof area. If your car rolled over or moved sideways, it would change the position of the air pocket. This is what happens when you swing, rock, or take the baby for a ride in the car. You put him in an inclined car seat, then you move: starting, stopping, and turning. This relieves the pressure points of the air pockets and gives temporary relief. Usually, when you stop the car, the baby will start crying again. This is an expensive way to get your baby relief; however, desperate parents do desperate things. Be cautious, though. Swing your baby gently and make sure the baby's head is supported because if you swing too aggressively, a baby's head and neck could be injured. Also, only operate a vehicle if you are fully awake and not too sleep deprived. Driving tired is the equivalent to driving drunk.[5] And, when taking a car ride, always place your baby in the proper car seat for his or her size, no matter how short the distance.

## Sucking

Babies find relief in sucking. "Sucking has its effects deep within the nervous system and triggers the calming reflex and releases natural chemicals within the brain," says Karp.[6] The nervous system controls everything; however, I believe that the major effect of sucking stimulates the digestive system and helps move the bowels. This is why your baby wants to eat all the time because sucking relieves the baby to some degree. However, over feeding eventually aggravates the problem because the excess milk causes too much pressure in the stomach. With the intense abdominal pressure pushing up against the stomach and diaphragm, the pain actually increases, which is also the major reason for the spit up and projectile vomit.

The easiest way to diagnose whether your baby is truly hungry or in pain is to offer a pacifier. If the baby sucks vigorously on the pacifier and then spits it out, he is probably hungry and can be offered a bottle. But if he is in extreme pain, he may also reject the pacifier because the sucking is not enough to relieve his pain. Many health experts recommend not introducing a pacifier until a baby and mom have an established breastfeeding relationship. This might be difficult for colicky babies, though, as these babies usually have a hard time latching on because of pain. Most babies I have seen who have used a pacifier during my treatment have no trouble switching from nursing to pacifier and vice versa.

**Other simple strategies**

Dr. Karp's 5 S's are great strategies to keep in mind when your baby is suffering. Through all his strategies, there is a theme of movement and change: Moving the baby and changing what the baby is experiencing. A warm bath, a warm bottle on baby's belly, or a massage are also popular suggestions. A warm bath changes the environment of the baby and could stimulate the bowels, same with a warm bottle and massage. But I have also seen a baby comforted by a mother's singing voice or playing a video from a cell phone. These aren't "fixes" and aren't in any way connected to alleviating the digestive system, but they are familiar and give comfort.

**Special Equipment**

Carrying on with the theme of motion are studies that encourage moms to walk with their babies[8] and have skin-to-skin contact.[9] Again, the motion can help move gas to relieve any pain, and the nearness to mom stabilizes the infant's heart rate and cements the bond between mother and baby. The mother's body temperature may also be like a heat pack on the baby's tummy, further reducing pain. For generations, moms have been strapping their babies on to accompany them throughout their daily routine. But if a baby is in severe pain, just being near mommy may not be enough. A study examining whether or not increased carrying time during the day would decrease symptoms for colicky babies reported that there was no significant change.[10] However, if baby wearing is an ideal bonding experience for you and your baby, there are some things to consider. Like swaddling, hip dysplasia is a health risk when using baby carriers, but there are many safe options available.

Another piece of equipment I see parents spend money on is anti-colic bottles. These bottles and nipples are designed to reduce the amount of air that babies swallow. These bottles are generally more expensive than basic bottles. And, although I have dealt with many babies who have colic, there is no significant difference between colicky breastfed, bottle-fed, or anti-colic bottle-fed babies.

**So, let's review.**

Some of the more helpful strategies include Dr. Karp's 5 S's which include swaddling, side or stomach positioning, shushing, swinging, and sucking. Although these aren't lasting solutions for colic, they are great methods for soothing. My caveat for swaddling is to be careful not to swaddle too tightly, as it has ramification for hip development and can add pain for a colicky baby. Hip dysplasia is also a concern when using baby carriers or slings. Do your research before using one.

Another consideration is whether babies should sleep on their stomachs or backs. The American Pediatrics Association recommends babies sleep on their back. However, I think this may still need more research, especially for colicky babies who may spit up when they sleep.

Above all, as stated in the previous chapter, my biggest advice is to use common sense when calming your baby. If you listen and watch your baby carefully, your baby will tell you exactly what he or she needs.

## Testimonial

Our first born, Harper, arrived in December 2008. When she was four days old, she began very long, intense periods of crying in the evening. She was inconsolable, restless, and seemed in pain. We suspected colic, and after visiting with our doctor, she confirmed that we were correct, but that there was nothing she could do to provide relief. It became a dreaded routine every evening to settle myself into

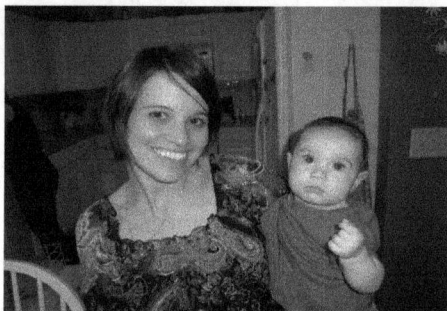

the rocking chair with my daughter, and prepare to just hold on for the duration of the crying, which typically lasted from 6pm to midnight. When we heard about Dr. Scharenberg, we were eager to meet with him to see if he could help. Our daughter was about 6 weeks old, and we felt sleep deprived, stressed, and anxious. Dr. Scharenberg agreed that colic seemed to be the cause of Harper's symptoms, and explained to us how he could help with daily treatments.

We were guardedly optimistic; it seemed too good to be true, but we were hopeful that with treatment we would see some improvement. We went to see Dr. Scharenberg five times a week for three weeks, and with each visit we would notice an improvement in Harper's symptoms; shorter periods of crying, longer periods of sleep, and in general a happier, less fussy baby.

After three weeks of treatment, we were amazed with the progress that was made! We were able to enjoy our baby, as she was happy, able to sleep better and no longer in pain. The service Dr. Scharenberg provides by offering these treatments is a valuable resource, and a great source of hope and encouragement for parents of babies who suffer from colic. We are forever grateful for the assistance he provided.

Crystal Jones

## Chapter 5: How Do I Tell if My Baby is Hungry or Hurting?

### *The ins and outs of baby body language*

**My Story**

Raising a baby in this day and age can be scary. The world is often negative and people are unhappy. Many are unsure why they are even here. With my ten to twelve-hour work days, I don't have a lot of down time, but when I do, I like studying the psychology of how thoughts control behavior. What interests me the most is how people keep positive attitudes toward life.

I always have a pile of books that I am reading. I read with a pen, underlining what sticks out to me, and I write my thoughts in the margins. I keep all the books I've read because I like to re-read them. I read through the passages I've highlighted and let them really sink in.

From what I've read and experienced in life, I found that one way to stay positive is to do the things you love. I think I know why I'm here, and I choose to use the knowledge I've gained to help others. It is my greatest joy to educate parents on how their baby is communicating with them, even without words.

**Understanding Body Language**

Communication can be described as actions, sounds, and behaviors that express the feelings and emotions of a living being. Communication is divided into three areas:

1. Body language - 55%

2. Tone of voice -  38%

3. What we say - 7%

If this is true, then when we learn to interpret what body language is, then we will know at least 55% of what the person is trying to tell us. When it pertains to a baby, what we have to do is realize we only have two lines of communication because they cannot express through words what they are feeling. Once you realize how important body language is and that it truly is telling you something, then to assume that your baby is fussy for no reason doesn't really make much sense.

**Body Language**

If a baby is crying, there has to be a reason. There are two main reasons a baby will cry. The first reason is that the baby has some physical discomfort, whether it is pain, like a headache, or just an uncomfortable feeling, like lying too long in one place. There could be many reasons; however, if any of these occur, the body language will tell us two things: where the pain or discomfort is and how bad it is.

If there is pain, it will cause the baby generally to move. To interpret the baby's actions, watch closely to what is moving and then watch to see if the motion is fast or slow. If the baby is showing full body motion, it is in pain. Like the following:  excessive kicking; movement of the whole body, torso, or arms; arching of the back; scratching at the face; pulling at ears and hair; and/or a hard abdomen. If the pain or discomfort is mild, the motion will be slow. If the movement is fast and much more aggressive, the pain level is much greater. If the pain is mild, the baby's eyes will be somewhat open or completely open. If the pain is more severe, then the eyes will be squinted or tightly closed. The baby's face will be round and red. He or she will be breathing faster and much more forcefully, causing an increased heart rate and increased respiration.

The second reason a baby will cry is if he is hungry. Is hunger pain discomfort? Let's say a teenager did not eat for over 24 hours. If for some reason he couldn't communicate via words, how would he communicate? He would probably bend over and flex his torso. He would probably groan or make noises, and the noises would be in proportion to how hungry he was.

When a baby is hungry, it will produce very similar body language. The motions will be more in the upper torso, arms, and head. The baby's legs will not kick as fast or as hard as they would if there was a lot of pressure in the intestines (like excessive gas). If the baby is hungry, the motion is localized in the upper body. Arms will be moving but not as stiff and severe as you would see with abdomen pain. The back will not arch as much; the head will not go back as with abdominal pain. The baby may smack her lips or show her tongue. There won't be scratching at the face and ears, and the baby won't be pulling his or her hair.  A simple key to remember is the more intense the hunger, the more body language you will see.

### Tone of Voice

The second form of communication is tone of voice. This is 38% of a baby's communication. There are two distinct cries: one is for pain, the other is for hunger.

If the baby is in pain, the cry is a distinct pattern of highs and lows. Imagine if you were experiencing severe pain. As you would scream out, the volume of the scream would change according to how often you felt the surge of pain. If the pain oscillated, then your yell would resemble ocean waves or the teeth on a saw blade, which would account for the highs and lows of your tone of voice. If the pain was very severe and didn't seem to let up, then you would give a long, loud scream.  In babies, this scream sometimes appears as if they aren't breathing. This is a scary for parents.

If a baby is hungry, usually the volume and pitch are more monotone than a painful cry. The pitch of a hungry baby's cry may be high or low, but usually the pitch and the volume will stay constant instead of increasing and decreasing.

There are times when your baby is hurting and also hungry. This makes it more difficult to read the body language and determine the tone of voice cry because there are two reasons for the body language and two different types of crying.

One way you can determine this would be to try to feed the baby. If the baby is only hungry, it will latch on, suck, and usually stay latched until becoming satisfied. If you attempt to feed the baby and they latch on fast, suck fast, but won't stay latched on, then you know the crying is due more to pain than hunger. This is where the body language of root and suck comes in. If the baby is in pain, they will continually detach from the nipple and then suckle back on. The cry will be loud, and the pitch and volume will both increase.

Sucking is helpful for a baby in pain because it stimulates the bowels and moves gas, taking the tension off the intestines. The pacifier can become a great diagnostic tool through this process. Offer the pacifier to the baby by holding the pacifier next to the baby's mouth. If the baby takes the pacifier, they just want to be comforted. The baby will not take the pacifier if they are hungry or in extreme pain.

When you offer the baby a pacifier, do not force it into their mouth. Just hold it next to their mouth. They will happily accept it if that's what they want. If they take it and then spit it out, they probably are hungry. If the baby spits it out and is still crying, they could be hungry or in extreme pain, or both.

During my colic treatment sessions where I strengthen the baby's ileocecal valve, I hold the baby and watch the baby's body language. As I am strengthening the valve, the bowels usually move, making the baby hungry. As I am feeding with a bottle, I will also offer the pacifier, switching back and forth depending on the baby's needs. In this way, I do not overfeed. If the baby is satisfied, they will continue to suck on the pacifier and might fall asleep. If they want more milk, they will spit out the pacifier, and I'll give them more milk.

I also encourage moms to try burping the baby by rolling the baby out flat on their back and then back up, like doing a sit up (while supporting the baby's head). This moves the gas around and sometimes releases extra built up pressure.

Please remember to always be patient and do things slowly. Offer the pacifier several time as the baby has to get use to the feel and taste of the pacifier. Don't be in a hurry. Let the baby make the decisions. If you do what the baby wants, you will be right.

If you do what you think is right, it probably won't work out as well. Being in a hurry always increases your stress level. Do everyone a favor and relax. Being stressed is never helpful for anyone.

How important is it to learn body language and tone of voice? It is extremely important because you will not only be able to help your baby more by understanding his or her needs but also so you don't do any harm.

**So, let's review.**

There are two main reasons a baby cries: discomfort or hunger. There are many different reasons why a baby could be uncomfortable, and there are different levels of discomfort, including the intensity of pain. A baby will react depending on the degree of discomfort. If there is pain, a baby will move its body forcibly for more pain and less forcibly for less pain. Their eyes will be shut tight, and their face will be red. Breathing will be harder and faster. They might arch their back, scratch at their face, pull at their ears or hair, and/or have a hard abdomen. The cry will have a distinct pattern of highs and lows. The cries could oscillate, like the ocean waves, as the pain increases and decreases, or it could be a long, loud scream for more intense pain. **PAINFUL CRY = Varying Volume + Varying Pitch**

The second reason a baby cries is hunger. The baby's body movements will be mostly in the upper torso, head, and arms. They might arch her back or throw their head back, but it won't be as intense as when they have abdominal pain. Their cry will be steadier and have a monotone volume and pitch.  **HUNGRY CRY = Monotone Volume + Monotone Pitch**

Sometimes babies are both hungry and painful.

**What we say**

Caregivers can communicate their frustrations and elations. They can speak words others will understand, but as we learned above, words are only 7% of how we communicate. It is the body language (55%) and tone of voice (38%) that does most of our communicating for us. That's why it is so important that we learn to read the body language and tone of voice of our babies. Because if we don't, no one else will communicate their needs. We are their words. And, they have a lot to say if we will only watch carefully and listen.

Every baby is a little different, but the more you study a baby, the more he or she will tell you exactly what he or she needs and wants. It won't happen instantly, but with patience, you'll be able to understand how your baby communicates.

## Testimonial

Dena was colicky from the day she was born. We had to have her sent into the hospital's nursery so we could get some sleep on the day she was born. She would fall asleep in my arms, but the second I put her down, she would scream. Being first-time parents, we looked to my parents and siblings for advice. I was told to try gripe water and Colic Calm.

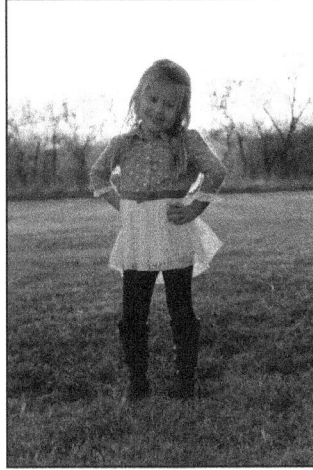

Both seemed to work for a day or two, but things would just go right back to 'normal.' When people would suggest my baby girl had colic, I would, for some reason, get very defensive (even with my husband). I felt that if she had colic, it would somehow reflect a failure on my part.

I still remember the day that I gave in to my husband's suggestion of taking Dena to Doc (he had heard about him from a few guys at his work and had been pressuring me to look into him). She had been crying almost all day long, and I just couldn't mentally take it anymore. At first I was scared of the thought of a chiropractor; I thought he was going to adjust my baby, and I was so relieved when I found out that was not the case. My husband and I were constantly at each other, and we were both just flat out exhausted. I called Doc's office and they scheduled us in that day (she was 2.5 weeks old). We first took her to her pediatrician for her scheduled 2-week appointment before heading to Doc's. She did agree that Dena had colic but never gave any suggestions on what to do.

Our first visit with Doc was a long one. It didn't take much time at all for him to determine that she not only had colic, but she had a bad case of it. We saw Doc just about every day, sometimes twice a day, for 2 weeks. I never strayed from the diet, but Doc did have to modify a few things to make it work better for us.

What stands out the most to me is our flight to California when Dena was 6 weeks old. Both my husband and I thought it was going to be a disaster. It turned out to be perfect. Many people came up to us after every flight to comment on how good our baby was. Our family will forever be thankful for the help we received from Doc.

Mom: Jennifer Eimers

# Chapter 6: Why Train Parents?

## *How educating parents does the greatest good*

### My story

My greatest reward is when the treatment is done, and parents are so appreciative and thankful. Parents go through a tremendous amount of stress and many tell me that they had given up on having more children until my colic treatment. In many ways, it changes their whole perspective as a parent. It enables them. They can do this big job of parenting. Their emotion at the end of the treatment is what makes it worth it for me. That's why I spend my weekdays and sometimes even my weekends treating babies. But, even with all the babies that I have treated, I still don't think it is enough. I want to enable parents to treat their own babies.

### Why do I want to teach parents to treat their own babies?

The reason we are teaching the parents instead of the doctors is because we want NO shortcuts. I was taught in chiropractic college many ways to treat adults, but I never had any classes on how to treat digestive problems in babies. Due to my love for children, I have spent hours and hours studying to find a way to treat colicky babies. I have succeeded, and I am ready to share this with the world. As I was contemplating how to do this, I initially thought the best way was to create educational seminars to teach other chiropractic physicians how to do this. But then, after a few meetings with colleagues, problems arose. The main problem was that this technique works, but you have to spend more time with each patient than would be done in a normal office setting. For example, many of my patients have to be seen at my house at odd hours of the night if they can't sleep due to severe pain. To find doctors who are willing to donate time and not charge a high fee for this could be challenging. The same is true with nurses or any other health care provider. Soon I realized that three things would happen:

1. The doctor would cut the time of the treatment.

2. The cost per treatment would go up.

3. The results of the treatment would go down.

My desire and intention is to teach people how to do this treatment and still retain my high level of success. After much thought, I decided to do a survey of the mothers whose babies I was treating and see if this might be something they would be interested in learning. In interviewing these parents, I found that mothers were excited to do this themselves. They repeatedly said, "Sign me up!" After thoroughly reviewing this new scenario, I realized it should be taught to the parents for a few reasons.

1. They are with their baby all the time.

2. They would take the necessary time to do this treatment because their love and commitment to their baby is higher than anyone else.

3. If their baby has crying spells in the night, they can treat the baby right away, letting it go back to sleep without pain.

4. They can treat the condition in half the time it would take me because they can treat the baby several times per day as opposed to one time per day, four to five times per week.

5. They will save a lot of time because they won't have to be going to the doctor's office every day for two weeks.

6. They will save money because there will be no more trips to the doctor and no more medicine.

7. When they have their next baby, they will have the treatment available, and they can start a preventative

treatment instead of waiting for the colic to develop and get worse.

8. The parents will have peace of mind that they can help their baby and take care of their own health (no more sleep deprivation due to sitting up rocking a crying baby to sleep).

9. The baby will be much healthier. It will gain weight, develop, and grow as it should instead of having a slow development.

10. If colic can be treated as a baby, the chances of digestive problems later will be reduced.

These are some of my main motivators for sharing this treatment with parents. The treatment works, but it is also challenging for parents because as caregivers, they do not want to do any harm to their child. They may be worried about doing the treatment themselves and hurting their baby. The first treatment session may take over one hour. The biggest problem will be continuing the treatment while the baby is kicking and crying and trying to get away. You will want to stop the treatment session, pick your baby up, calm him down, and start over. Your thoughts may be,

"Am I doing it wrong? Does this really work?" If you do stop the treatment session, you will lose all that you have gained. The muscle has to have time to strengthen. If you study and learn everything I am trying to teach you before starting the treatment, this will encourage you to stay the course. When parents do not fully understand what I am sharing, they become skeptical about the treatment, and they do not have the faith to stick with it. When done correctly, the treatment will reduce colic symptoms. I have seen this case after case. (Read the testimonials at the end of every chapter.)

**Possible struggles**

Moms, in particular, have a hard time listening to their babies cry. They want to console them and may feel that by not consoling them, they are a bad mother. Moms have heard and may have dreamed about the special bond between mother and child. However, as a mom recovers from childbirth, she may be sleep-deprived, charged with hormones, and discouraged. Some moms suffer from having what has been dubbed the "baby blues." For many, this is more than just a feeling of being "blue." Although less common, postpartum depression and postpartum obsessive-compulsive disorder are real struggles for new moms. According to the U.S. Department of Health and Human Services, 13% of pregnant women and new moms have depression.[1] Authors Shoshanna S. Bennett and Pec Indman describe it well in their book *Beyond the Blues: A Guide to Understanding and Treating Prenatal and Postpartum Depression*. They write the following:

> Perinatal (during pregnancy and postpartum) mood disorders are caused primarily by hormonal changes which then affect the neurotransmitters (brain chemicals). Life stressors, such as moving, illness, poor partner support, financial problems, and social isolation are certainly also important and will negatively affect the woman's mental state. Conversely, strong emotional, social, and physical support will greatly facilitate her recovery.[2]

Even moms who do not have depression may be frustrated with being unable to comfort a colicky baby. Although desperate for a solution, a skeptical mom may start this treatment but be unable to successfully finish because of her baby's cries. The false belief that the treatment is creating more pain for the baby coupled with the desire to console the baby instead of completing the treatment are big

hurdles for moms.

| **What can a mom do if she is feeling this way?** |
| --- |

- First, know that you are not alone. Many moms feel this way. Talk to your obstetrician, your partner, and other people in your support system about how you are doing. Sometimes more professional help is needed, and that is okay.
- Secondly, take care of yourself. Get some sleep. Eat a good meal. Giving birth and taking care of an infant is difficult, especially a colicky infant. Let others help so you can rejuvenate and heal.
- Thirdly, change your expectations. Understand that, although a beautiful time for your family, having a baby is also very stressful. Don't expect to have it all figured out.

Fathers, also, may have difficulty staying strong with this

treatment. In general, dads do not have as much patience as moms.

Dad will try to console the baby but will give up quickly and give the

baby back to the mother, which is what mom also wants. A father

may take this personally and feel like the baby is rejecting him.

Fathers usually have the attitude of "it will be okay if they cry it out,"

which, for babies with weak ileocecal valves, could mean hours and hours of crying until they fall asleep from exhaustion.

Another discouragement for parents is when the symptoms re-occur during the treatment. From the first treatment session to the last, you will see recurring symptoms which make you think the colic symptoms are returning. Stay with the treatment for as long as it takes, whether it is 10 or 20 treatment sessions. If you stop the treatment, you lose, and most of all, your baby will lose. It is always better to do the treatment longer to be certain. You won't be doing harm by doing more, but you can do harm if you stop too soon.

Our society is not a patient one. We want instant food, instant service, and instant result. But just like any weight loss plan, the more patient you are in keeping with the treatment, the better the results in the long run. Think about going to the gym. When you start your New Year's resolution on January 1, the first day is painful. Your muscles are not used to the new regiment, and they scream for you to stop. After you finish, you feel accomplished, but you may be sore and tired. The second day of your new workout is probably the hardest. Your muscles are sore and are not yet used to the strain you are putting on them. If you give up, your muscles will not have any change, but if you continue, they will start to strengthen, adapting to your new routine.

Your baby is also strengthening a muscle. The ileocecal valve is a muscle between the small and large intestines. The first and second treatment sessions are usually the most difficult because the muscle is learning how to work properly. But, if the caregiver endures through those first treatments, there are immediate results with fewer severe crying episodes.

The other time parents are vulnerable to discouragement is halfway through the treatment. Let's go back to the New Year's resolution analogy. If your goal was to lose weight, you may have lost a lot of weight at first, and then your progress reaches a plateau. The same seems to occur with the colic treatment. The colic symptoms might stay the same or some may even return halfway through the treatment. This is where your patience is of the utmost importance. If you stop now, all the progress you've gained may be lost. This is especially true with the colic treatment. If you stop before the muscle is completely strengthened, the digested milk will continue to seep back into the small intestine, causing pain and inflammation. This, in turn, will bring the colic symptoms back.

So what should a caregiver do to avoid these pitfalls? First, read this entire book. Study and learn everything you can about my treatment. Believe that the treatment will work for your baby and your family.

Secondly, before you start the treatment, write your goal. Why is this treatment important to you? How will it improve your baby's and your family's lives? Strategize. Having a colicky baby drains you emotionally. When you are starting to have doubts, where will you find your motivation? Who can you turn to for encouragement? Let the people in your life who are your support team know about the treatment. Let them know you will need their encouragement. At the end of this chapter you will find a few inspirational quotes reminding parents and grandparents how powerful and influential they are. You are the difference in your child's life.

**So, let's review.**

My goal is to treat thousands of babies with colic symptoms, eliminating the risk of shaken baby syndrome and giving both the family and the baby a better quality of life. The treatment is easy to learn, and there are a lot of reasons this treatment will be very helpful for you, your baby, and your family.

There are also some drawbacks to treating your baby yourself, including your own fears. But, there are ways to combat that fear including being well informed and finding motivation prior to starting the treatment.

Please take this seriously. It will work for you; however, you must be patient, and you must do it correctly. It is extremely important that parents use patience when treating their babies. If you want the treatment sessions to work, take no shortcuts. The reason we are teaching parents instead of doctors is because we want NO shortcuts.

## Words of Inspiration

**For Moms**

"Successful mothers are not the ones that have never struggled. They are the ones that never give up, despite the struggles."

-Sharon Jaynes

"To the world you are a Mother, but to your family you are the World." -Author Unknown

"Being a mother is learning about strengths you didn't know you had, and dealing with fears you didn't know existed." -Linda Wooten

"Sometimes the smallest things take up the most room in your heart."

-Winnie the Pooh

**For Dads**

"Any man can be a father, but it takes someone special to be a Dad."

-Anne Geddes

"The quality of a father can be seen in the goals, dreams and aspirations he sets not only for himself, but for his family."

-Reed Markham

"A good father is one of the most unsung, unpraised, unnoticed, and yet one of the most valuable assets in our society." -Billy Graham

"A dad is a son's first hero and a daughter's first love."

-Author Unknown

**For Grandparents**

"Grandchildren give us a second chance to do things better because

they bring out the best in us." -Author Unknown

"Nobody can do for little children what grandparents do.

Grandparents sort of sprinkle stardust over the lives of little children."

-Alex Haley

"A grandchild fills a space in your heart that you never knew was

empty." -Author Unknown

"Grandparents, like heroes, are as necessary to a child's growth as

vitamins." -Joyce Allston

**See the goal worksheet at the end of the book to help you put into**

**words your own motivations and goals before treating your baby.**

## Chapter 7: What is the Ileocecal Valve?

### *An explanation of the digestive anatomy and the generalized idea of treatment*

**My story**

With my chiropractic practice up and running, I continued to see a number of colicky babies and was determined to help them. As I spent hours and hours treating babies, things started to click. There were certain things that would help the babies improve. With patience, I learned from each baby I worked with. There were specific reactions I could predict. Every patient was different. It was the common-case babies who taught me the colic treatment. As a young man starting my practice, time was on my hands. This is what I learned.

Colic is not the rule of three.

If colic isn't corrected, it can go on with varying digestive symptoms the rest of a baby's life.

In most cases, colic is caused by a weak valve between the small and large intestines. This muscle is called the ileocecal valve. Babies' valves are not immature muscles but weakened muscles that need to be strengthened by my colic treatment.

This treatment is time tested. It is not a massage treatment, soothing technique, or a chiropractic adjustment. This technique is unique from all other colic remedies advertised. I have seen it eliminate the digestive pain of babies (into adulthood) if understood and performed correctly.

## The GI tract

When a baby comes into my office, the colic diagnosis is made by the consideration of the baby's health history and a physical exam. It cannot be diagnosed by lab or x-ray exams. Parents usually mention that their baby has been diagnosed or it has been suggested by medical professionals that the baby has acid reflux. Colic is completely separate from acid reflux or gastroesophageal reflux disease (GERD); however, most of the time colic is confused with, or misdiagnosed as, acid reflux. The symptoms are similar, but, like mentioned earlier, most acid reflux cases are actually colic.

So what is happening internally to cause colic symptoms? It all starts as baby eats.

As soon as a baby swallows milk, the digestion race has begun.

The GI (gastrointestinal) tract is the path the milk takes from mouth to diaper. Although there are many other factors involved in digestion, including the nervous and circulatory systems, the main body parts involved in the process are the mouth, esophagus, stomach, small intestine, and large intestine. These body parts work together to break down the consumed food and drink into nutrients of carbohydrates, proteins, fats, and vitamins. These nutrients are carried throughout the body and help baby grow. The first year of a baby's life sees the most drastic developments. Babies are expected to triple their birth weight by the time they are one-year-old.[1] That is a lot of growing!

The mouth starts the digestion process by chewing the food. For a baby, it is less chewing and more swallowing. The act of sucking and even swallowing is a skill babies have been practicing since in utero; although, newborns and preemies sometimes have difficulty swallowing. Once in the esophagus, the milk encounters a muscle between the esophagus and stomach called the lower esophageal sphincter. It is the gatekeeper. The muscle relaxes and lets food pass through to the stomach. This is an involuntary action started by the act of swallowing and controlled by the esophagus and brain.

The upper stomach muscles relax to accept the milk from the esophagus, and the lower stomach muscles mix the milk with the digestive juices, creating something called chyme. This continues on to the small intestine.

The small intestine continues the digestion by mixing the milk with digestive juices from the liver, pancreas, and intestine. The walls of the small intestine absorb the nutrients and send it through the bloodstream to the rest of the body. Once the food comes to the large intestine, all the nutrients have been absorbed and all that remains is waste. The large intestine takes the waste, absorbing water and any leftover nutrients, and turns it from liquid to solid. The waste stays in the rectum until it is pushed out by a bowel movement. Diaper duty.

The valve between the small and large intestine is called the ileocecal valve. It is meant to be a one-way road, only allowing the digested food to go from the small to the large intestine. However, if the valve is weak, it can create leakage, much like a backed up pipe. The small intestine then begins digesting the material again. This creates severe increases in flatulence (gas), putting pressure inside the small intestine and causing distention to the intestine, which results in pain. This leads to all the other symptoms identified as colic.

So, although soothing techniques may temporarily ease the pain caused by the leakage, nothing can help colic except strengthening the valve.

By strengthening the ileocecal valve, the valve will stay closed and only open for digested food to move from the small intestine to the large intestine, as it is meant to do. Like strengthening any muscle, patience is essential. Using a specific technique so that no harm is done to the baby's digestive system, the ileocecal valve is strengthened through several treatments.

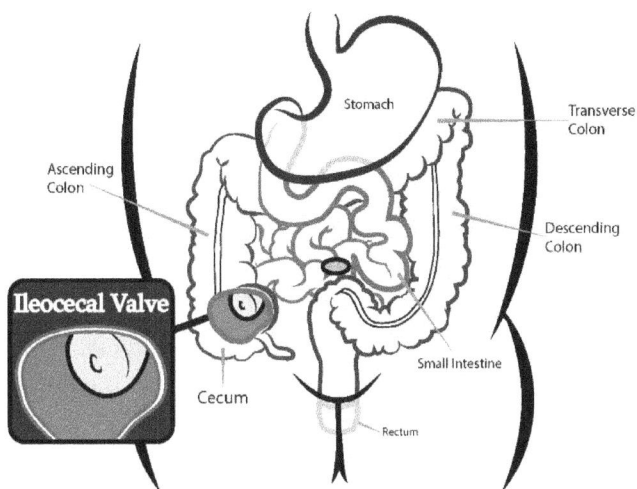

**Colic treatment**

On average, the baby's first treatment session is one to two hours long. Moms report that after the first treatment session, their babies show 20-30% improvement. I continue to see the baby every day for about two weeks, depending of the severity of the colic symptoms. Each treatment varies on the amount of time, but the treatment sessions generally become shorter as the valve is strengthened.

If the treatment is stopped before the valve is completely strengthened, then the digested milk will continue to leak back when the valve doesn't close properly. If treatment isn't continued, then the leakage will steadily weaken the valve, bringing back colic symptoms and erasing any progress made. It is so important to be patient with the process, just like you would be if your goal was to gain muscle mass at the gym. Repetitive, consistent work will strengthen your baby's ileocecal valve with time.

When babies are treated in my office, I have parents fill out a detailed survey on their baby's symptoms including crying times, sleep, etc. They also give me a percentage of improvement. Sometimes parents ask me what I would give the baby, but I never tell them what I think because I don't want them to finish the treatment too early and rush the results. As the baby's caregivers, parents spend more time with the baby and are able to assess the baby's symptoms better than I could within the hour long visit. I don't release the baby until the improvement is satisfactory to the parents, not just based on what I think. If I agree with the assessment, then I release the baby. If I don't agree, I keep treating the baby until I feel the baby is ready. But, most of the time, parents' assessments are the same as mine.

The data I have collected from hundreds of parents has helped me see how the treatment typically progresses. Included at the end of this book is a similar survey to help you keep your own log. The first couple of treatment sessions are usually the longest and produce the most drastic improvements. Let's go back to the New Year's resolution at the gym. When you start working out, you immediately feel the effects of using and working your muscles. You might shed the pounds easily. The feeling is great, and you are pumped to continue this new routine.

During the middle of the treatment (usually around treatment session 6 or 7), there is a plateau with only small improvements. At the gym, you might get discouraged that the drastic changes have slowed down. Likewise, parents sometimes get skeptical and want to quit during this time. They may even see a regression. But, like stated above, it is important to keep doing the treatment. Even though the improvements are slight, consistency is important.

Near the end of the treatment sessions, the improvement continues, but it is not as drastic as when the treatment sessions first started. This is also true at the gym. If you push through your plateau, then the consistency of your routine will show through the loss of a pound or two until you hit and maintain your ideal weight. The number of treatment sessions depends on the severity of the colic. While most babies respond well to 10 treatment sessions, more severe cases might require more. You cannot hurt your baby by continuing the treatment if you are unsure, but you can cause your baby to regress if you stop the treatment too soon.

**So, let's review.**

When a baby swallows milk, the milk travels through the mouth, esophagus, stomach, small intestine, and large intestine. Then, it's time for a diaper change. In most cases, colic is the result of a weak ileocecal valve between the small and large intestines. The valve is supposed to keep the digested milk on the one-way path to the large intestine. However, if the valve is weak, the digested milk seeps back, causing severe flatulence and thus pressure and pain on the small intestine.

The key to stopping this is to strengthen the ileocecal valve. This is done through my colic treatment. These treatment sessions are not a massage, spinal adjustment, or soothing technique but a gentle, time-tested technique that will improve the baby's digestive health for a lifetime.

The number of treatment sessions varies depending on the severity of the colic, but generally there are around 10 treatment sessions. The first treatment session is usually the longest from one to two hours. Subsequent treatment sessions are shorter. There is a survey at the end of the book to help you log your baby's personal progress. Also, the videos that complement this book show the step-by-step process on how to do the treatment sessions.

The decision to treat your baby will have short-term and long-term effects. In the short-term, your family will be able to bond and enjoy your baby's precious early years. The discouragement and desperation you once felt will make way for adoration and confidence. Adoration for every smile and new milestone your baby makes and confidence in yourself to understand your baby and be able to help your baby grow into the adult he or she was meant to be. In the long-term, the risk of digestive problems will be greatly reduced, as untreated colic turns into adult digestive disorders.

The decision to treat your baby requires dedication and patience, but it will be the best decision you can make for your baby and family.

## What I consider before starting treatment on a baby

- Age of the baby--Is the baby old enough to be teething? This is also a painful process.
- Bottle or breastfed--If the baby is bottle-fed, he could be constipated from the added iron in the formula. Are his bowels moving? If the baby is breastfed, the mother's diet could be contributing to the weakening of the ileocecal valve.
- Diagnosed with any other health issue-- Sometimes colic can be coupled with another illness.
- Any recent injury or fall--The birthing process is tough on babies and can result in injury. Also, many babies fall before they turn one. These are things to consider.
- On any medicine or had any recent vaccines-- Most medicines have adverse reactions. Although they are uncommon, I always ask about this. Also, vaccines sometimes cause adverse reactions. Once again, only a small minority reports reaction, but it's still something to consider.
- Fever--Does the baby have a fever? This is uncommon, but if a baby does have a fever, it usually means he is fighting an infection.

As all babies are unique, I take all the answers into consideration when diagnosing and proceeding with my treatment. For the most part, babies can be treated for colic even if they are struggling with another illness. In some cases, it may even help speed up the recovery of the other illness.

## Testimonial

We brought our son, Tyler, to Dr. Scharenberg for colic treatment when he was five weeks old. Tyler had been displaying signs of colic since coming home from the hospital. He would scream, eat, and occasionally sleep. He wanted to nurse around the clock and was constantly spitting up, including multiple bouts of projectile vomiting a day. He was having problems gaining weight and was starting to miss the typical milestones you would expect of a baby his age. His screams were so loud and persistent that our neighbors could hear him crying in the middle of the night from their bedroom.

Our pediatrician did several tests to rule out serious conditions, including pyloric stenosis before diagnosing our son with acid reflux. The doctor prescribed a medication that hopefully would help with the condition. When filling the prescription, the pharmacist strongly cautioned us about the possible side effects in a child as small as ours. Around the same time, my OBGYN had provided us with information on Dr. Scharenberg and suggested we investigate, as several of her patients had positive experiences with the doctor's colic treatment.

We did research on Dr. Scharenberg and his treatment. While reviews online were overwhelmingly positive, my husband and I were both skeptics and thought there was a good chance the treatment was a crock and the results all hype. However, as any parent with an extremely colicky child will confirm, you're willing to try almost anything to help your child. The screams of pain they wail are enough to rip your heart out. We decided, as the treatment was noninvasive, we would delay the medication (and its possible side effects) for a very short time and try Dr. Scharenberg's treatments.

During the first visit, Dr. Scharenberg explained his theory on the cause of colic, described the history of how he developed his treatment, and laid out his plan of action for our son. While his explanations seemed plausible, we were still skeptics. However, after the end of the first session, our son was more relaxed than we had ever seen him and he slept for nearly three hours following that first treatment. He slept through the night for the first time and the next day, smiled for the first time.

Progress was fairly consistent after that. While we had ups and downs and days where it seemed as if we were regressing, the overall improvement was noticed by everyone who had seen our son before we began the treatments. His projectile vomiting disappeared and our fussy, screaming child was transformed into a happy, smiling baby whom we could actually enjoy. We were able to get some sleep, go out in public, and develop some resemblance of a routine.

Dr. Scharenberg was great with Tyler and extremely patient with our questions, concerns, and skepticism. He let the treatment speak for itself and always took the time to listen to any issues we had throughout the process. The decision to visit Dr. Scharenberg was the right one for our son and family and our only regret is not having found him sooner.

Mom: Bobbi

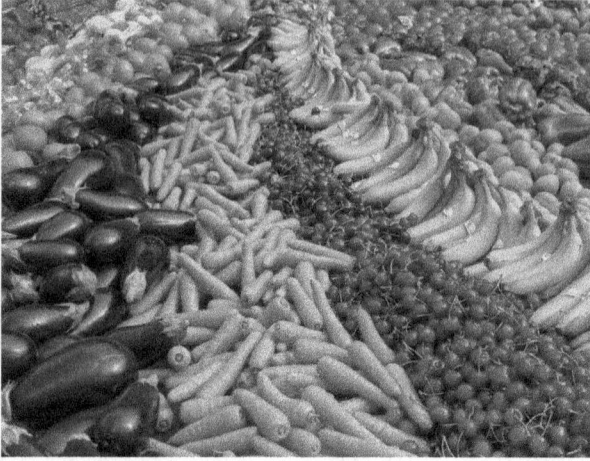

## Chapter 8: Does Diet Affect Colic?

### *The different approaches to breastfed vs. bottle-fed babies during*

### *Treatment*

**One mom's story**

Sarah just always assumed she would breastfeed her baby. She didn't even read any literature or take the class offered at her local hospital. Her mother assured her that it was a natural event. Sarah had been nursed so she knew that's what she wanted for her baby. But, as her week-old baby cried with red face, she wondered if it was the best choice for both the baby and herself. Sarah was sore and exhausted. She wasn't sure if there was something wrong with her milk supply. Was her baby latching on correctly? Is breastfeeding right for every new mom?

**How to feed a baby who has colic**

Should every mother breastfeed? The obvious answer would seem to be yes; however, there are many circumstances in which the mother simply cannot. Whether it be for health reasons, medication, alcohol, a conflicting occupation, or maybe the mother simply can't produce enough milk to satisfy the baby, breastfeeding isn't always an option. If a new mother is healthy and there is no physiological reason why she can't breastfeed, then it only makes sense to give the baby the most natural food possible, as it contains many beneficial components, such as hormones, which are not present in formula preparations.

However you feed your baby, it is important that you adjust your baby's diet, if needed, to help the healing process. Colic is a condition that affects a baby's intestines and is affected by the milk that a baby drinks.

## Feeding techniques

It is important to distinguish between a babies' hunger and pain cries (as discussed in a previous chapter). Once you know when to feed your baby, you should follow these two important tips:

1. Feed baby only when hungry, not in pain.

2. Stop feeding when baby is satisfied.

## Feeding breastfed babies

There are various factors that could cause or contribute to a colicky situation, including what a mother eats while breastfeeding. Breast milk can have an effect on the baby, which can exacerbate colic symptoms. The first thing to look at is the mother's diet. What I have found through working with hundreds of moms is that certain foods can weaken the baby's ileocecal valve, which lies between the small and large intestines. This weakening is what causes, in most cases, colic symptoms. Certain high fiber or protein foods will weaken this muscle, as a result increasing leakage (and colic symptoms). These foods are also harder to digest, which creates a higher production of intestinal gas. There are other substances such as spices, carbonated beverages, caffeine, herbs, and even vitamin supplements (especially with iron) which aggravate and create more leakage and gas production.

How would you know if you are eating a food that is making your baby worse? See the suggested list of foods below and follow these helpful tips in combination with my colic treatment to make the road to recovery much quicker.

The "foods you can eat" list below isn't necessarily a healthy diet, but it has shown to work the best until the colic has been corrected. Usually colicky babies are doing well after eight to ten treatment sessions. If the baby is asymptomatic, I usually start the mother back on hamburger. If this works well for about two days, we slowly start adding foods back into their diet and within two to three weeks moms can usually go back to their normal diets without causing any colic symptoms.

If the mother eats something on the NO list before the baby is ready, the baby will have a negative response at the first feeding. It takes twelve to twenty-four hours to get the "NO food" out of the mother's system to stop bothering the baby. There is no way to determine in advance which foods will bother the baby, so I suggest the mother only eat what is on the YES list until the baby's colic is corrected.

Mothers have told me that it is hard to follow the diet; however, they have also told me how it is a small sacrifice as the colic symptoms subside. If a mother doesn't follow the diet, the baby is the main person who suffers. In turn, everyone else around will suffer too because the baby will go back to crying. If the mother eats food on the NO list, which weakens the valve, it will take longer to correct the colic, and it will take more treatments to alleviate the pain and symptoms.

| Foods to Avoid | Foods you can eat |
|---|---|
| **Types of Protein to avoid**<br>Pork<br>Beef | **Types of Protein you can eat**<br>Chicken<br>Turkey<br>Fish |
| **Types of Vegetables to avoid**<br>Tomatoes<br>Broccoli<br>Cauliflower<br>Celery<br>Asparagus<br>Lettuce<br>Spinach<br>Onions<br>Peppers<br>Squash<br>All beans except green beans | **Types of Vegetables you can eat**<br>Carrots<br>Green beans<br>Corn<br>Potatoes<br>Peas |
| **Types of Fruit to avoid**<br>Bananas | **Types of Fruit you can eat**<br>All fruit except bananas |
| **Types of Grains to avoid**<br>Rice<br>Nuts<br>Whole Wheat<br>Pasta with sauces and garlic | **Types of Grains you can eat**<br>Plain white bread (try to avoid a lot of yeast)<br>Tortilla<br>Plain pasta<br>Macaroni and cheese<br>Cheerios<br>Oatmeal<br>Crackers |
| **Types of Dairy to avoid**<br>(Most dairy okay to eat. Although not a dairy, avoid eggs, which can be found in the dairy aisle.) | **Types of Dairy you can eat**<br>Milk<br>Cheese<br>Plain or vanilla yogurt<br>Cottage cheese<br>Butter<br>Sour cream<br>Ice cream |

| Beverages and Sweets to avoid | Beverages and Sweets you can eat |
| --- | --- |
| Chocolate | Vanilla ice cream |
| Caffeine: pop, coffee, & tea | Vanilla pudding |
| Carbonated beverages | Honey |
| Alcohol | Vanilla wafers |
| | |
| Spices and Condiments to avoid | |
| All spices, especially cinnamon | |
| Smoke flavoring | |
| Garlic | |
| Ketchup | |
| Mustard | |
| Pickles | |
| Mayonnaise | |
| | |
| Avoid all Mexican Food and Italian Food | |

If the mother doesn't change her diet, can the treatment still correct the colic? Yes, but it will take many more treatments and will take longer in general. Remember, high fiber foods and high protein always make it worse. Also, lettuce and celery seem to be the worst for weakening the ileocecal valve.

If you are still having issues after following the diet, read the ingredients of what you are eating. For instance, a patient of mine was eating a certain cereal each morning, only to find out later that the small trace of nuts hidden in the ingredients was causing problems. Also, granola bars are hard to find without rice, crushed nuts, or cinnamon. Look for eggs in the ingredients, while also watching for food like turkey bacon, as the smoke seasoning could make colic worse as well. Any special seasonings you use when grilling or cooking usually contain some form of garlic or dried onions, making them potential colic-aggressors. Don't overlook what's on your sandwich, as mustard and pickles could aggravate colic as well as mayonnaise, which contains eggs.

If your baby is doing well after eight to ten treatment sessions, you can start reintroducing foods into your diet and find what foods work best for both you and your baby. The best way to find all your "yes" foods is to go back to the basics and add one food in at a time, seeing how it reacts to your body, your baby's body, and even checking for allergies. Most mothers report being able to eat the bulk of the "no" list with the exception of chocolate and caffeine within two to three weeks after completion of treatment. I know. Parents have told me that those are the two must-haves for sleep-deprived moms, but for some reason, babies don't react well with the caffeine. It may be several weeks before you can reintroduce those into your diet. Add each item in slowly and watch for a reaction.

Follow these guidelines for breastfeeding mothers, and your whole family will be happy you did. See the end of the book for two-weeks of meal and snack ideas.

**Feeding bottle-fed babies**

Bottle-fed (formula) babies bring with them a different issue. The baby's diet does not change; however, all formula contains iron. What does iron do? It hardens and stiffens the fecal material and causes constipation. Since the baby is already having intestinal problems and has excessive gas, it becomes very painful for a colicky baby to move its bowels.

A breastfed baby will normally move its bowels during nursing or right after; however, a bottle-fed baby is lucky to have a bowel movement every twelve to twenty-four hours. Many parents are told by their doctors that it is okay for a baby to go three and even up to five days without a bowel movement. My experience shows that a baby with more frequent bowel movements will respond faster to treatment, and the colic can be alleviated much sooner. If the parent helps move the baby's bowels at least every twenty-four hours, the speed of recovery is much faster, and the baby doesn't have to suffer near as long. There are a couple of ways to help the baby move its bowels.

1.  You can use a rectal thermometer and periodically stimulate the rectum to increase peristaltic activity of the intestine.

2. You can use pediatric infant suppositories to help move the fecal material through the intestines.

Parents ask, "Won't my baby become dependent on these and make it so they have to be used all the time?" I would say if you are doing the colic treatment as recommended, this will help move the bowels better and more frequently, and since colic is usually corrected in about two weeks, they will not become dependent in such a short period. It is so much better to help the baby move the bowels than it is to make them struggle, cry in severe pain, and aggravate the umbilical hernia. Also, the parents don't have to watch their baby suffer as much. One of the worst things young parents have to endure is watching their baby scream and cry and not be able to help them.

There are a lot of home remedies for moving the bowels, such as adding Karo syrup to baby's milk or apple juice. Will this hurt the baby? Will it work? As long as you do no harm, it might be worth a try. Be careful not to use anything toxic or anything with alcohol when trying home remedies. Please remember that there are always side effects to drugs, so be very careful and diligent when making decisions to administer medicine. Lastly, there are low-iron formulas which may be a better fit for you baby. One that many patients have used with success is Similac 60/40. It is not usually stocked in the pharmacy, but you can order it online.

**Satisfying hunger pains and avoiding spit up and projectile vomit**

When a baby cries, you can determine if a baby is hungry or in pain by observing his or her body language and tone of voice. If the baby is hungrier than in pain, the baby will latch on and suck hard and fast until he or she begins to feel satisfied. What is actually happening to make the baby feel satisfied? Is it how much milk is in the stomach? No, it has to do with blood sugar levels.

Appetite is controlled by blood sugar levels. Think about how you feel when you know your blood sugar is dropping. Several symptoms can occur.

1. You begin to feel fussy or irritable.

2. You start feeling a sensation in the stomach and the intestines. Have you ever experienced your stomach growling?

3. Your emotions begin to change. You feel more anxious. You now begin to focus more on eating and less on what you are doing or saying.

4. Your tone of voice can change.

5. You may get a weak or sick feeling in your gut.

6. You start noticing cravings, many times the hungrier you get, the more you begin to crave foods high in sugar and fat.

Babies can go through all of these same symptoms. Now think about how you feel when you see food. Do you become more anxious? Do you become more aggressive? What happens when you finally get some food?

You may stuff your mouth full, chew faster, swallow faster, and usually eat more than if you had eaten earlier. One question often debated: Is it better to eat six healthy, smaller meals or three full, large meals? The answer may depend on the person, but dieticians will agree that it is important not to let your blood sugar get so low as to create a situation where you risk overeating or eating out of control. Babies are similar. Why does blood sugar go up and down? It is not only caused by the types of food we eat, but also by the amount. It is also affected by everything else that is going on in our bodies. Not only is the pancreas producing the hormone insulin to help regulate our blood sugar, but other hormone producers such as the thyroid, adrenals, and endocrine glands are constantly in flux. This is true not only within the baby's body, but if the baby is breastfed, then the mother's hormones are also affecting the baby.

Think about what happens when the blood sugar goes too low. We usually eat too fast, too much, and don't stop in time for the blood sugar to level off. So what happens in the case of the baby? Remember, being satisfied isn't dependent on the volume of food consumed, but is regulated by the blood sugar. So, if the baby eats so much that the stomach is full of milk (and if there is a lot of pressure against the stomach from the bloating of the large and small intestines), then there will be pain, which causes crying. Parents also may not burp the baby very well and eventually the baby will projectile vomit. Parents wonder why the baby keeps spitting up after he or she is done projectile vomiting, and the answer is that there is just too much milk in the tank (stomach).

The keys to stopping projectile vomiting and spitting up are:

1. Relieving the pressure in the intestine.

2. Feeding the baby only when he is hungry.

3. Stop feeding when the baby slows down.

4. Burping the baby regularly.

5. Giving the baby a pacifier, after they have been satisfied and he will go to sleep.

6. Not putting the baby on a regular feeding schedule (like 3 ounces every 3 hours). Listening to the baby's body language and tone of voice for cues for when they are hungry instead.

7. Being aware of the previous feeding with amount and time.

We don't always get hungry at the same time or rate. Hormones regularly affect blood sugar, so the baby will vary in how much they eat and time between feedings. Don't expect the baby to eat the same all the time. However, some babies may get hungry around the same time to form a routine.

Learning your baby's cues and following the above guidelines can be challenging at first but will get easier as you and your baby settle into a comfortable pattern. They will give you signs that they is hungry, and you will be able to feed them before letting their blood sugar drop too low.

**So, let's review.**

What are some of the things to keep in mind when feeding your baby?

Whether you breastfeed or bottle-feed, the biggest tips for feeding a colicky baby are:

1. Feed baby only when hungry, not in pain.

2. Stop feeding when baby is satisfied.

Breastfed babies are unique in that anything their mom eats, they also receive. High fiber and protein foods that the mom eats weaken the baby's ileocecal valve, which creates re-digestion and irritation in the baby's digestive system. It is important that while the baby is receiving colic treatment, the mom sticks to the strict diet explained in this chapter. Although the food list is not necessarily a healthy diet, moms report that they can slowly re-introduce food into their diet after 8-10 treatment sessions. They can eat everything on the NO list within two to three weeks of completion of treatment.

Bottle-fed babies are challenged with iron-rich formulas which causes constipation. Changing to a low-iron formula, like Similac 60/40, benefits bottle-fed babies. As for dealing with the constipation, you can use either a rectal thermometer to periodically stimulate the rectum and increase peristaltic activity of the intestines, or use pediatric infant suppositories to help move the bowels. Although some parents worry this could be habit forming for babies, it is important to help the baby move his or her stools at least once every twenty-four hours. When the treatment is complete, babies will have an easier time doing it themselves.

Whether a baby is breastfed or bottle-fed, there are a few tips to avoid spit up and projectile vomit. Like mentioned above, the most important tips are:

1. Feed baby only when hungry, not in pain.
2. Stop feeding when baby is satisfied.

Other tips include burping the baby regularly, giving the baby a pacifier when he is satisfied (slows down eating), and watching baby for cues when he is hungry instead of putting him on a regimented feeding schedule.

A baby will be satisfied, not by the amount of milk given, but when his blood sugar levels stay balanced. Keep learning your baby's hunger cues to know when and how much to feed them, not inadvertently overfeeding or underfeeding them.

**See the feeding log at the end of the book to help record your baby's milk intake.**

## Testimonial

At 3 weeks old I took Paisley to see Dr. Scharenberg in desperate need of help. I had an extremely fussy baby and nothing helped. I could tell she was in pain and unable to do anything to console her. Dr.

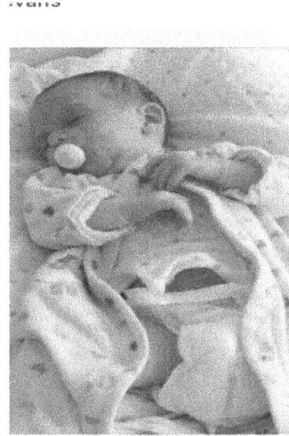

Scharenberg scheduled us right away and examined her little tummy and told me that she did have mild colic. Dr. Scharenberg wanted to see Paisley every day until her symptoms subsided. Every day for 3 weeks I took her to his office and within the first appointment the difference was amazing. At every appointment she improved and was such a relaxed baby. By the end of our 3 weeks she was content and happy with no tummy troubles. She took her feedings without screaming and was sleeping through the night. We are so thankful he was recommended to us and I continue to recommend him to people needing help with their babies.

-Kaycee Reynolds

## Chapter 9: Is My Baby Getting Enough Milk When I Breastfeed?

*Some common breastfeeding problems and solutions*

**My story**

The hardest thing I discuss with moms is if the milk they are producing is enough for their babies. Many times moms will breastfeed their babies, but for some reason, the babies are not receiving enough milk at that time. This is particularly emotional for moms, as the ability to breastfeed has been linked to motherhood for many generations. The following is information that has helped many of the mothers whose babies I have treated and includes the following: how breastfeeding works, possibility of baby having lip and/or tongue-ties, producing too little or too much milk.

**How breastfeeding works[1]**

As soon as a mom becomes pregnant, her body starts preparing to breastfeed. Pregnancy hormones of estrogen and progesterone cause breasts to grow and start to prepare the inner highway for milk. This is also what causes breasts to feel uncomfortable during the first few months of pregnancy.

Breasts are composed of nerves, blood vessels, and tissues. There are four types of tissue in the breast: milk glands which produce milk, milk ducts which carry milk, supporting tissue which gives structure and shape to breasts, and protective fat which cushion the breast from injury. It is the amount of protective fat which determines the size of a breast. Milk production is not dependent on the size or shape of a woman's breasts. Most women have enough glands to produce milk, no matter the size.

The milk production starts as soon as the baby is born. After the placenta is delivered, the estrogen and progesterone that were so high in pregnancy decreases. The hormone prolactin, which is already high in mom's system and is also the hormone that causes the uterus to contract during and after labor, helps mom release milk.

When a baby sucks on the breast, the nerves in the breast signal the brain to release hormones that make and eject the milk. These hormones are prolactin and oxytocin. The more a baby nurses, the more prolactin will be released and more milk produced. When oxytocin is released, it causes the tiny muscle cells surrounding the milk glands to contract. This expels milk and fat globules out of the milk glands and into the ducts, and it allows the milk duct to propel the milk through the duct system by stimulating muscle cells that line the duct system. This is also known as the "let-down reflex."

The first milk mom produces is called colostrum. It is a thick, sticky milk that is high in salt, protein, and immune components. It is lower in milk sugar lactose and fat content, which makes it the perfect fit for baby's new digestive system. It is also full of antibodies, white blood cells, and other immune properties which protect the baby from infection.

Approximately two to four days postpartum, "milk comes in" and the colostrum milk becomes a transitional milk. Every day the composition is different. The volume is steadily increasing, as well as the fat and lactose. The protein, on the other hand, is decreasing.

Mature milk comes in after ten to fourteen days. Its composition is consistent, except the fat content varies with what is known as foremilk and hindmilk. Foremilk is the "first" milk in the nursing session, and it is low in fat, around 2%, and watery. The hindmilk is after the milk let-down, also known as the "let-down reflex." This milk is 10% fat or higher. When the baby reaches six months, the protein in the milk drops, and this is usually when babies are introduced to solid food.

As a baby grows, they will need more and more milk to nourish them. If a mom can't successfully drain the milk she is producing at the beginning of breastfeeding, she will have difficulty producing enough later on. The amount of milk produced is based on the amount removed. Milk production will maintain as long as milk continues to be removed. Although this book is not able to fully explore these issues, some common reasons for impaired milk removal to be aware of include infrequent or short feedings, flat/inverted nipples, breast infections, sore nipples, breast engorgement, or a baby's tongue/lip tie. Sometimes the baby might be going through the motions of feeding without getting a full feeding because milk doesn't let-down or the mom is not producing enough milk.[1]

## Tongue/Lip-ties

If babies have completed my colic treatment and are still having problem breastfeeding, sometimes it is because of a tongue or lip-tie. Tongue or lip-ties (known as ankyloglossia or Tethered Oral

Tissue) are malformations common in infants but can be easily missed by professionals who aren't trained to look for them. These ties are connecting tissue that restricts the tongue or lip or sometimes cheeks from the full range of motion needed for feeding.

Some babies have both tongue and lip-ties. Others may have one or the other. Lower lip-ties and cheek ties (called buccal) can also occur, affecting jaw and dental development, breathing, chewing, swallowing, and digestion.[2] They can also impair speech development later on and can be a big problem for breastfeeding. Blogger Heather Dessinger, better known as Mommypotamus, says it well: "a mother's breast can come in many different sizes and shapes, as can a baby's mouth. The crucial factor is how the two function together."[3] If a baby has a tie, then it makes it even more difficult for mom and baby to work together.

The common procedure for correcting a restrictive frenulum is called a frenectomy, where the restricting tissue is cut. Moms have reported immediate results in better breastfeeding with their infants after the frenectomy. But, I have also seen babies who continue to struggle after the frenectomy, not because the procedure was unsuccessful, but because the babies are colicky and are having

problems feeding due to high pain levels. They need my colic

treatment.

### Baby's Symptoms
- Babies may not be able to stimulate milk production through vigorous nursing, leading to low milk supply
- Painful nursing/early weaning because child gets too frustrated
- Improper tongue mobility may prevent babies from clearing milk from their mouth, causing tooth decay (especially in the front teeth)
- Sleep deprivation for mama and baby (due to the need for frequent feeding)
- Speech difficulties
- Gap between teeth/ Jaw issues

### Mom's Symptoms

- Creased /flat/blanched nipples after feedings
- Cracked/blistered /bleeding nipples
- Discomfort while nursing
- Plugged ducts
- Thrush/Mastitis
- Sleep deprivation (Because baby is not able to nurse efficiently they compensate by nursing more often, leading to frequent night feedings.)

One of the front runners for ankyloglossia is Dr.Lawrence Kotlow, DDS. Here is a list of compiles problems and symptoms he has compiled.[3]

### Problems Associated with Tongue and Lip Ties

- Difficulty latching on or falls off the breast easily
- Gumming or chewing the nipple while nursing
- Unable to hold a [pacifier] or bottle
- Gassy (babies with ties often swallow a lot of air because they cannot maintain suction properly)
- Poor weight gain
- Excessive Drooling
- Baby is not able to fully drain breast
- Choking on milk or popping off to gasp for air while nursing
- Falling asleep during feedings, then waking for a short while later to nurse again
- Sleep deprivation (due to the need for frequent feedings)
- Extended nursing episodes- aka marathon nursing sessions
- Clicking noises while sucking
- Popping on and off breast often
- Biting (Babies who have trouble grasping the nipple sometimes try to use their teeth to hold on.)
- Gap between teeth/jaw issue

**Producing too little milk**

Some of the moms I work with have babies who continue to cry during colic treatment, not because of pain, but hunger. For some reason or another, the mom may not be producing enough milk during that nursing session. This could be because the baby wasn't drinking fully before the colic treatment because of pain and now when the baby is able to consume more, the mom's production hasn't caught up to the demand. Or, it could also be due to various other reasons. I tell moms to offer a couple ounces of milk in a bottle after the nursing session. If the baby drinks it readily, chances are that mom may not be producing enough milk during that session.

This is tough for moms to hear, but it doesn't mean she needs to give up nursing all together. There are several things that she can do to help.

1.  Don't stress. Stress can impede the breastfeeding process. Think happy thoughts about how you are nourishing your baby and be in a comfortable position, whether that be in a chair, lying down, etc. The more you can be in a relaxing position

that is comfortable for both you and baby, the better. Also, don't neglect sleep. Lack of sleep can contribute to stress.

2.  Be sure the baby is latching on properly. If you are having difficulties, get help from a lactation consultant sooner versus later. Milk is produced because milk is removed. If baby isn't latching on and is having difficulty sucking, then the milk won't be drained, and mom won't be able to produce the milk as baby grows. The sooner you can ensure the latch is correct and baby is getting milk, the sooner milk is removed and more milk is produced.

3.  Nurse often. Newborns will want to feed 8-12 times a day.[1] And when baby isn't nursing, pump. Some moms pump after a feeding to make sure all the excess milk is removed and keep the pump on even after all the milk is released for a few minutes. The stimulation will encourage the milk glands to produce more next time by showing a demand.

4.  Eat well. Breastfeeding takes a lot out of moms. Make sure you are eating at least 500 additional calories to make up for how hard your body is working. I also like to recommend the

herb fenugreek to increase milk flow. Some say blessed thistle and alfalfa work well when taken with fenugreek.[4] Also, these foods are said to increase production: oats, brewer's yeast, flaxseed, hummus, papaya, spinach, carrots, asparagus, salmon, and apricots.[5] Yeast, spinach, and asparagus can weaken the valve and cause more flatulence or gas. I suggest not using these until the colic is relieved.

5. Lower your expectations. If you need to supplement breastfeeding with bottle-feeding, that's okay. Your baby is getting fed and is growing. That's what's important. Many moms are worried that if they give their baby a bottle, he or she will no longer want to nurse. I've seen several babies who switch back and forth with no problem. This is also a chance for dad or another caregiver to feed baby and bond in a new way.

**Producing too much milk**

I would never tell a mom she is producing too much milk, but sometimes moms say that their breasts are engorged or their let-down is overactive. Here are some suggestions.

Moms who complain about breasts being painful or feeling too full may have engorged breasts. This is a sign that the breasts are producing more milk than the baby is drinking. This is especially common four to six weeks postpartum as the milk production is adjusting to what baby needs. The risk is that babies could be drinking too much foremilk and not enough hindmilk, which helps sustain them between feedings and gives them the fat they need to grow. On another note, this can be very painful for mom. A simple solution to this is to pump before feeding. Many moms do this and save or donate the milk they produce. But, with this, because the milk is being removed, the breasts will continue to increase production. Another option is using a cold compress to try and relieve the pain. Or, some of the suggestions below for an overactive let-down may help with engorgement, as they are usually connected.

An overactive let-down can be frustrating for both mom and baby. If baby is choking, pulling away, or having a hard time keeping up with the milk flow, there are a couple things you can do.

1.  Pump before feeding. This can take some of the initial

    pressure off the feeding and none of the milk is spoiled as the pumped milk can be saved. Or, if you are worried about continuing to produce too much, only have baby nurse on one breast per feeding. At the next feeding, have baby get any hindmilk left on that breast before switching to the new breast. This is called block feeding.[6] Be careful not to wait too long between feeding, though, as the breast that wasn't drained can become engorged and painful.

2. Feed reclined or lying down. In this way, gravity is against you, and when the letdown comes, it won't come rushing down into baby's mouth and may be more easily controlled.

3. Pull baby off at let-down. The first let-down is thirty seconds to one minute into the feeding session. This is usually the most powerful one. Catch the milk with a towel or milk storage bag. Once the let-down is done, continue to let baby feed like normal.

**Give yourself grace**

Whether breastfeeding is meeting your ideals or has become more like a nightmare, allow yourself some grace. Baby is new at this. And if you are a first-time mom, you are new at this, too. If you are an experienced mom, every baby is different, and you may feed this baby differently than your other babies. The important thing is that you are doing the best you can to ensure your baby is being nourished. That could mean that you nurse and then have another caregiver give your baby a bottle. Whatever it looks like for your family, know that it doesn't take away from what you can offer as a mom.

For dads and other caregivers, keep encouraging and helping mom in whatever ways you can. Having a newborn come into the family can be challenging for everyone. Suddenly there is an addition to your family who is completely dependent. This can be exhilarating and exhausting. Although you may not be the main source of nourishment for the baby, there are plenty of ways you can be a part of the breastfeeding process. Keep that mom fed, offer to do a bottle night feed to give her some rest, encourage her when she's frustrated. She may be the one nursing, but she needs the support of others to sustain her.

**So, let's review.**

A mom's body starts preparing for breastfeeding as soon as

she becomes pregnant. Although the shape and size of women's breasts are different, most women have sufficient milk glands to nurse. How much milk a mom produces is linked directly to how much milk is being removed. There are various reasons for having trouble removing the milk. They include infrequent or short feedings, flat/inverted nipples, breast infections, sore nipples, breast engorgement, or a baby's tongue/lip tie. Seeking help and seeing a lactation consultant sooner versus later is recommended, as the longer a mom waits, the more likely nursing will not be successful.

One problem sometimes missed by professionals is tongue and lip-ties. Tethered oral tissue is extra skin that restricts the tongue, lips, and sometimes cheeks from performing normally, especially limiting successful breastfeeding. The surgical procedure for correcting this is called a frenectomy. Mothers report that their babies have had immediate breastfeeding success after the correction.

Other common breastfeeding problems include producing too little milk or producing too much milk. For problems with producing too little milk, I recommend avoiding stress, ensuring a proper latch, nursing often, eating well, and lowering expectations. As a mother, you want to nourish your baby, but allowing a bottle feed while you are waiting on your milk supply, does not negate your motherhood. The important thing is that your baby is being fed. For moms with an active let-down or who complain that they are "producing too much milk," I suggest pumping before feeding, feeding reclined, or pulling baby off at let-down.

The most important piece of advice I like to give moms is to give you grace. Being a mom is physically demanding and emotionally draining. Allow others to help with your baby so you can take care of yourself and allow your body to work the way it was designed to. It's okay if you need to supplement with bottle-feeding. The important thing is that your baby is being fed and is getting the nourishment he or she needs to thrive.

## Testimonial

My husband and I already knew what colic was like after [our first child] Dena, so with Taylor we were extra cautious. After Taylor and I were released from the hospital, we made an appointment to have Doc look at her. She seemed fine, but we just wanted to make sure that if she did have colic, we caught it right away. At her appointment, Doc said that she was okay, but to keep an eye on her.

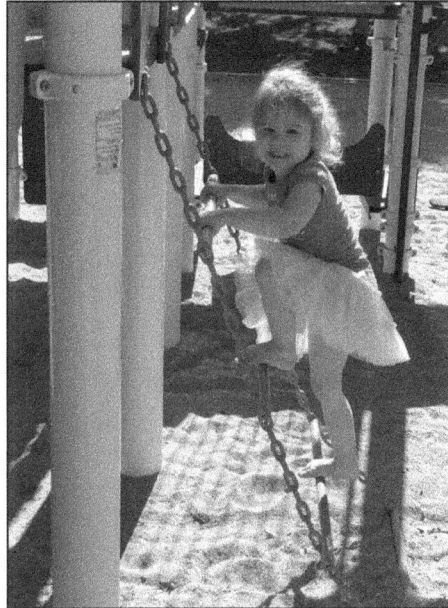

For the first 5 weeks, Taylor was the ideal baby, but starting at 5 weeks she started to show signs of colic. She started grunting, screaming, scratching and she was no longer pooping regularly. We only allowed the signs to go on for 2 days before we called and made another appointment with Doc.

This time when Doc checked her out, he said she did in fact have colic. He told us it was a very mild case, so the treatment would be fast. Taylor was only treated 5 times and honestly probably only needed 4 treatments. Since her treatment was so quick, we never had a period where things seemed to get worse. Every day was an improvement.

Mom: Jennifer Eimers

## Chapter 10: Frequently Asked Questions

### *What parents most want to know*

Below is a list of questions to help you review what you have

learned in this book and a few topics that were not covered in depth.

These are some of the most common questions I receive before,

during, and after giving babies the colic treatment.

**What is colic?**

Colic is a diagnosis given for babies who cry excessively. The

historic marker for colic is when a baby cries for three hours, three

days a week, for more than three weeks. See Ch. 1 for more

information on the history of colic. Sometimes the reason a baby cries

is because of an illness; however, a majority of the time it is because

the baby's ileocecal valve is weak and needs strengthening.

See Ch. 2 for more information on different illnesses.

**Is there a solution for colic?**

Although the medical community will tell you there is no fix

for colic, I have used my colic treatment to treat babies with weak ileocecal valves and have seen parents completely satisfied with the results. See Ch. 7 for an explanation of how my colic treatment works.

**How can I tell if my baby has colic?**

There are many symptoms associated with colic. Check out Ch. 1 for a full list of colic symptoms.

**How long does colic last?**

Babies with colic turn into children and adults with digestive problems if not treated. Very rarely does colic correct itself.

**Is acid reflux colic?**

Both acid reflux and colic are misunderstood. Many times colic is misdiagnosed as acid reflux. See Ch. 2 for more information about the differences between colic and acid reflux.

**Could my baby's cries be something other than colic?**

In most cases, colic is the result of a weak ileocecal valve; however, sometimes a baby's colic symptoms could be the result of something else. Or, it could be an illness coupled with colic. See Ch. 2 for a list of other possible reasons your baby could have colic symptoms.

**Should I keep giving my baby gas drops or gripe water during the**

**colic treatment?**

The goal of my treatment is for babies not to be dependent on any chemical substances. Parents report that gas drops and gripe water only temporarily relieve their babies' symptoms. In some cases, it could be contributing to the weakening of the ileocecal valve and causing the colic symptoms, which is why I tell parents not to use it during the treatment. See Ch. 3 for more information on gas drops and gripe water.

**Do soothing techniques work for colic?**

Some soothing techniques are good to comfort your baby. There are other strategies promoted that are not overly helpful. See Ch. 4 for an explanation on today's most popular soothing techniques and strategies.

**How can I tell if my baby is in pain or just hungry?**

Even though babies cannot talk, they still have a lot they can tell us through their body language and tone of voice. See Ch. 5 for more information on distinguishing between a hurting cry and a hungry cry.

**Why aren't other health professionals using this technique?**

After discussing my work with a couple of colleagues, I realized that the amount of time needed to perform my treatment was too long for a typical office visit. Due to the long hours needed, there were a couple things that would end up happening. Either the cost would become so high that many parents could not afford the treatment or the treatment time would be minimized, resulting in higher reoccurrences of colic symptoms. Patience is the key to the treatment. The only way I foresaw the treatment's continued success would be to take the treatment directly to parents. Parents already spend long periods of time with their babies, and they are the ones who would do anything to rid their children's pain. It only made sense to teach parents the colic treatment. See Ch. 6 on why train parents.

**What is the colic treatment?**

After much study and research, I developed a technique that strengthens the valve between the small and large intestines. This valve is called the ileocecal valve. With a lot of patience, this technique works to strengthen the valve and decrease the colic symptoms until they are gone. See Ch. 7 for a full explanation of the treatment.

## How long before the treatment works?

Parents report that their babies show improvements immediately after the first treatment. Parents see continued improvement after each sequential treatment, but keep in mind, the first treatment is the longest. The baby may scream and resist, but the first treatment does not hurt the baby any more than the pain he is already in. See Ch. 7 for more information on the treatment and see Ch. 6 on how to mentally commit to the treatment.

## Can I hurt my baby using this technique?

It is important that you fully understand the information given in this book and be fully dedicated to the treatment before starting it. If done correctly, this treatment works precisely and does not hurt the baby. Your baby is already in so much pain, and it should be a comfort to know that the treatment does not add to your baby's pain, but it will ease it. I encourage you to read the entire book to help you understand the themes repeated throughout.

## How long do I continue the treatment?

When I perform the treatment in my office, the treatment is around ten sessions. I see the baby every day for two weeks. When the treatment sessions are able to be given more frequently, the duration will shorten. It is important not to stop the treatment too soon, as it would defeat any progress that has been made. See Ch. 7 for more information on the colic treatment.

**Does the treatment work if I breastfeed?**

Yes, the treatment works for formula or breastfed babies. When a mother breastfeeds, it is important that she follows my diet while the baby is being treated. This will speed the recovery for the baby. In most cases, the mom will be able to return to her regular diet after the baby finishes treatment by slowly reintroducing foods to see if the baby reacts. See Ch. 8 for more information regarding breastfeeding and treatment.

**What if my baby is constipated?**

Many formula-fed babies are constipated from the iron in their formula. I recommend changing formulas or giving infant suppositories to help regulate their system. In breastfed babies, I recommend mothers eat more fruit to help loosen the bowels. See Ch. 8 for more information regarding formulas and suppositories.

**Projectile vomit. Suggestions?**

Yes! Try not to overfeed your baby. Instead of feeding on a schedule or thinking your baby must drink a certain amount of milk, think of feeding as regulating your baby's blood sugar levels. Watch for signs of hunger. See Ch. 8 for more information on projectile vomit, and see Ch. 5 for understanding baby body language, which will help you know when your baby is hungry.

**Could my baby be teething? What are the signs of teething?**

I've had one family return to me post-treatment wondering if their baby had colic again. The baby was exhibiting some of the same signs of colic, but the baby was teething. Parents have told me that the best remedies for teething is teething tablets, a cold washcloth, or a hard teething toy to gnaw. Confused whether your baby is colicky or teething? See Ch. 1 for a full list of colic symptoms. Here are some of the signs of teething:

1. more than usual drooling
2. baby puts hands and fists in mouth
3. arching the back
4. putting the head back as far as it can
5. rocking the head back and forth

6. won't take pacifier

7. won't take breast or bottle

8. has a higher pitched cry (a scream)

9. puts fingers in the mouth over the sore tooth

10. body language and tone of voice doesn't match normal colic
    cry

11. continues to cry when fully fed

12. stomach may be soft but continues to cry

13. eyes may open or shut, depending on the amount of pain

14. legs and arms move different than with abdominal colic pain

15. back and legs may be stiff with head moving back and forth
    and usually a loud cry

**Could my baby be crying because of a vaccine?**

Vaccines may have adverse reactions. Before you give your baby a vaccine, be educated. Understand the disease(s) the vaccine covers and how common it is. Research what is in the vaccine and any adverse reactions the vaccine may cause. Talk to your pediatrician about the risks and benefits for your baby, and read the vaccine's pharmaceutical pamphlet. Research shows that only a small percentage of individuals have adverse reactions to vaccines, but if you suspect your baby is having an adverse reaction, contact your pediatrician immediately. If your baby is having difficulty breathing or is unconscious, contact your local emergency medical services immediately.

**Is my baby too old to be treated?**

The answer is no. I have treated toddlers, children, and even grandmas with weakened ileocecal valves. The symptoms from a weakened ileocecal valve differ depending on the patient's age, but they all are linked to digestive problems. The sooner a baby can be treated, the better. However, people can be treated at any age.

**How do I know if my breastmilk supply is enough for my baby?**

Sometimes a mom's supply is not enough to feed a baby. This is one of the hardest things to work through with a mom. Often a mom so desperately wants to nourish her baby, but she's just not producing enough milk. What I recommend moms do is to pump and see how much milk they are producing. Sometimes frequent pumping will increase the milk supply. In the meantime, the baby can be supplemented with the pumped milk, formula, or another mom's donated milk. If the milk supply never comes in, don't be discouraged. There are a multitude of options to keep your little one fed. For more information on the breastfeeding process, see Ch. 9.

**I want my baby treated! What's my next step?**

I am developing instructional videos, which are designed to train parents that complement this book. These videos will be available on my website in the near future. For more information on why I want to train parents, see Ch. 6. Or, if you'd like to work with me directly, contact my offices: Scharenberg Chiropractic Offices. I have treated babies from all the over the United States and abroad. My greatest desire is to rid children from this painful condition. Contact us today and see how we can help your family!

## Conclusion

In this time of rapid change, there has been very little help for babies with colic and very little progress in understanding crying babies. Although there have been many theories, products, and chemicals produced which claim to eliminate colic, most of these techniques and products have been helpful but not curative.

I know this because of my extensive experience working with the caregivers of colicky babies. I have spent the majority of my career researching, studying, and observing the information that I have given in this book.  It is my greatest hope that through this book moms, dads, and other caregivers will feel more confident when making decisions for their colicky babies. Colic does not need to be endured!

After helping colicky babies for forty years, I know my colic technique is a gentle and effective way of treating colic. What this treatment has truly taught me is patience. In this busy, face-paced world, patience is a virtue we sometimes lack. But learning this technique and having the patience to follow through is worth it for your baby, your family, and you. May God bless your journey!

For more specific information on the how to receive or learn

the treatment discussed in this book, contact Dr. Scharenberg:

**www.stoppingcolic.com**

**www.docscharenberg@gmail.com**

Wichita, KS 67206

This book is for educational purposes only and is not meant to diagnose or treat. The opinions offered in this book are that of the author based on his experiences of working with thousands of infants and parents.

All testimonials are a reflection of each individual's perspective of how the treatment affected their family.

## More Testimonials

I have three children. My oldest, Ariel, had severe colic

symptoms until she was 4-months old and continued to act

uncomfortable until she was a

toddler. We didn't know that there

was help out there for colic, so we

just suffered through the pain.

When my second child Eden was

born, she also began to exhibit colic

symptoms at about 10 days old. She

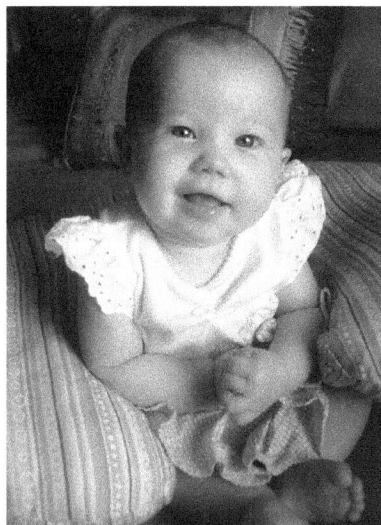

acted like she was uncomfortable and in pain constantly.  A friend had

referred Dr. Scharenberg to us, so we decided to try it.  I was nervous

about taking my newborn to a chiropractor, but Dr. Scharenberg's

technique doesn't involve spinal adjustment, and he was very helpful

in explaining the process, which set my mind at ease. I could instantly

tell that Dr. Scharenberg was very knowledgeable about colic and

colic treatment. He was extremely caring and kind with my baby. Doc

really was concerned about my baby's well-being and was going to do

whatever it took to make her feel better.

I saw a massive difference in my baby after just one treatment. Her stomach, which had been hard and bloated, now felt soft like it should. She began the treatment crying, and by the end she was fast asleep. She slept more soundly after that treatment than she ever had before. She was also able to lie on her back comfortably. It took a few weeks of treatments before she 'graduated' with no colic symptoms. The improvement was undeniable. After Doc had worked his magic, she became the happiest of all three of my babies. She slept the best, ate the best, and was content to just sit in her car seat or lay on the floor. I was so grateful to have the blessing of knowing Dr. Scharenberg. His colic treatment definitely helped improve the quality of life for my baby and also my family. If your baby exhibits any of the colic symptoms listed, then I HIGHLY recommend you schedule an appointment with the Doc. You will be so glad that you did!!!

Mom: Naomi Pinkston

***

My husband Nate and I had our first baby on May 9th of 2018. Our son was born a healthy baby but was born grunting. He would grunt and cry from having an upset belly. I felt so bad for him. He would sleep for maybe a couple hours at a time and then all he would do is eat until he went to sleep then wake up crying. When he was about 6 weeks old he spent a good 3 hours crying and I didn't know

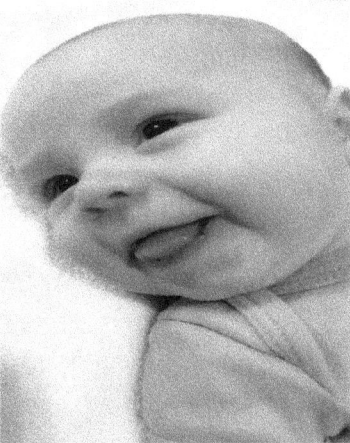

what to do any more. I tried everything from gas drops, to colic calm, to a warm bath, massaging his belly and so much more. Nothing would sooth him. I called Nate at 4:30 when he was about to be off work to see if he was on his way home and he wasn't. He was going to be late. By this point I was crying along with Daniel. Nate reminded me of someone suggesting to us to see this Chiropractor. I didn't really want to because I never saw a chiropractor for myself so why in the world would I allow my baby to be seen by one. I decided on that Wednesday evening to email Dr. Scharenbergs clinic to see what would happen.

Well, 7:30 the next morning Dr. himself gave me a call to check in on us after hearing we needed help with our little guy. He got us in on Thursday evening. Daniel went in crying and came out sleeping a good 4 hours after just his first treatment. That first evening Dr. worked on Daniel for a good 2 hours. He spent time talking to Nate and I about what colic is and what causes colic. He then shared with us how he could help us. After asking us if we would like him to help our baby, Dr. then proceeded to do the first treatment that evening. We ended up seeing Dr. 12 times.

Ever since that first treatment it's like we brought home a new baby. Daniel sleeps all night every night. I can count on one hand how many nights he has woke up in the middle of the night. It has usually been due to a bad dream. Daniel is able to rest so much better. He is a lot more comfortable. He doesn't fuss. He is a happy content baby now. I don't know what we would do without Dr. Scharenberg!

We are soooo thankful for not only treating our baby boy and his colic but the time he spent teaching us as new parents how to care for our baby boy. The whole staff in the clinic was so supportive and helpful during the time of the treatments. I recommend all parents to take their babies to Dr. if you are experiencing any problems with your little one. I know when we have another one we will be taking our next one to Dr.

I recommend for anyone who needs help with getting relief for their crying newborn baby that is dealing with colic to go see Dr. He is a blessing sent from above for our family! We can't thank Dr. enough for the love and care he poured into Daniel. He is now almost 5 months old and as happy as can be. I pick up Daniel from daycare and they are always telling me amazed they are at how relaxed Daniel is. I know it's because of the treatment Dr. gave Daniel. Thank you Dr. for caring for our baby boy so we can enjoy this time becoming new parents. We aren't scared now to have another one someday!!!!

Mom: Susan Dick

For three long exhausting and trying years, our daughter Claire was in an incredible amount of stomach pain. This pain consumed our lives. We tried everything from the time she was about three months old to three years old; diets when I was breastfeeding, changing formulas,

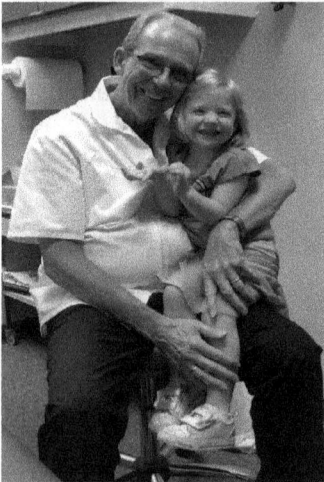

Mylicon, little tummies, Simetheicone drops, molasses, charcoal, Zantacs, Prevacid, elimination diets as she began eating foods, etc. On average, she cried twelve hours a day did not sleep much and when she did sleep she slept best on her tummy or side. She screamed in the car, ALWAYS. She was either constipated or had diarrhea. She would end up falling asleep sitting up in her crib because it relieved some of the pain when she was upright. She never used her swing, bouncer, or mamaroo because of the incline position. She screamed after eating, had lots of hiccups, spitting up, she picked at her ears until they bled when her tummy hurt, she was never relaxed, extended belly, and would scram so hard she would pop blood vessels in her eyes. We were in and out of the pediatrician's office and were always told it was colic and she will grow out of it. As she reached twelve months and never grew out of the colic the pediatrician wanted her on adult strength prevacid daily. We knew the long-term effects were not good but the pediatrician didn't seem worried. We went back to the internet searching for more answers. We saw a holistic doctor who was able to make life somewhat manageable but never took away the underlying problem, as it still caused her pain. The hurt in our hearts, constant anxiety and day to day exhaustion was getting unbearable. Constantly questioning what she ate, what it could be, do other kids act this way, etc.

My cousin saw Dr. Scharenberg on Facebook and immediately texted me. I was hesitant to call but we had nothing to lose, we could not continue living like this any longer. I received a phone call back from Dr. Scharenberg himself! He was confident and reassuring, so we headed to Wichita! He listened to us with our concerns and asked us questions, he truly cared about Claire and us as parents. He knew the stress weighed on us all. We met with him twice a day for one week as he massaged the valves that were weak causing this pain. After the third treatment, she was a new child!! A very happy, sweet, three-year-old who could eat, play, and sleep with no pain!! I kept waiting and waiting for a tummy ache because after three years of them it was weird not having them!!! They never came…. Our lives had forever changed all thanks to Dr. Scharenberg.

I wish we had known about him when she was a newborn! Dr. Scharenberg is passionate about what he does, he spends the time to help these babies and kids feel good inside. Claire still tells me months later that her tummy doesn't hurt anymore because Dr. S fixed it!!

Mom: Courtney Robinson

***

We didn't realize Imogen had colic or reflux until she was almost 2 months old. Every baby cries and spits up, so we didn't think too much about it. While at the Wesley Parent/Baby playgroup, one of the teacher/coordinators (a lactation consultant) suggested going to the doctor. After taking her in, she was prescribed Zantac, which was not the easiest to give to a baby. We had also tried gripe water at night too, when we couldn't get her to sleep. She would try staying up every night from midnight to 5 a.m. crying. A masseuse friend suggested going to see Dr. Scharenberg. She had taken her own baby to see him for colic and constipation. I wasn't sure it would help, but at this point we were in survival mode.

After the first week she was doing really well then the doctor left for a work vacation. Poor Imogen went backwards, though, not as bad as our first visit. After a couple of [treatments], she was back on track. I think she had 14-15 visits. The special diet was not easy to stick to especially when you tend to eat healthy or attend a holiday party. I was very happy to start re-incorporating foods but [was] able to track specific foods that would throw Imogen in a tailspin (now I know to avoid them completely if they cause an issue). Imogen still cries and even spits up occasionally like all babies... but she is doing good since seeing Dr. Scharenberg. Thank you so much!

Family: The Goodmans

***

My son was born May 2014 and promptly showed us he had healthy lungs. He would scream for hours in the evening. Diagnosis:

colic. As I started to look at the medical definition of colic, it didn't make sense that a baby would cry for no reason. And, I did not know how, as a new mom, I would be able to get through the allotted three months that my baby books said colic would last. So, I started doing my own research and asked everyone I knew what to do. My husband and I tried swaddling, shushing, swinging, and just holding the baby all night long.

Our pediatrician told us that he could hear gas in his intestines and gave us some home remedies that he said could be helpful. I proceeded to change my diet, since I was breastfeeding, and we invested in some gripe water and 7up. Someone mentioned to us the ileocecal valve (the valve between the large and small intestines), which I put into my ever growing list of what the problem could be.

Then, after a 2-hour photo session where our baby boy screamed the entire time, our photographer mentioned a chiropractor that worked with colicky babies. As I got on Dr. Scharenberg's website, all the pieces started to come together. It made sense to me that the milk that seemed to calm him momentarily was actually causing digestive havoc. And, on the website, Dr. Scharenberg talked about the same intestinal valve that was mentioned to me earlier.

I immediately made an appointment.

After only a couple sessions with Dr. S, I laid my son on his back, and he fell asleep within minutes, something that would have been a two-hour event prior. Dr. Scharenberg spent the time during our sessions to answer questions and educate me in the process. And after I felt confident that my son had made an 180-degree improvement, Dr. S graduated him: colic free!

Mom: Ashley Shannon

***

I am so thankful we were referred to Doc Scharenberg. Our little boy Justus was experiencing extreme grunting, hard tummy and constant fussiness. He had a constant need to suck but would not take a pacifier, therefore I had turned into a human pacifier and I was exhausted, my nipples were bruised and sore and my gut just kept telling me he shouldn't be in pain and it shouldn't be this hard! I tried everything from gripe water to bicycling his legs and after many sleepless nights of researching Doc's website I trusted my gut and made an appointment. I had a hard time admitting he had colic because he didn't have the typical crying symptoms I had been told about. Since we are over a two and half hour drive from Wichita he saw him two times a day for treatment. After the first treatment I could already tell a difference! Doc taught me about his different cries and as treatment continued Justus kept getting better and better. According to his big sister "brother found his happy" thanks to Doc. The week after we brought him home he slept in his crib, fell asleep on his own, took a pacifier, the grunting had significantly improved, I am no longer anxious to go out in public and he always has a smile on his face!! We are forever grateful to have found our happy as a family of four!

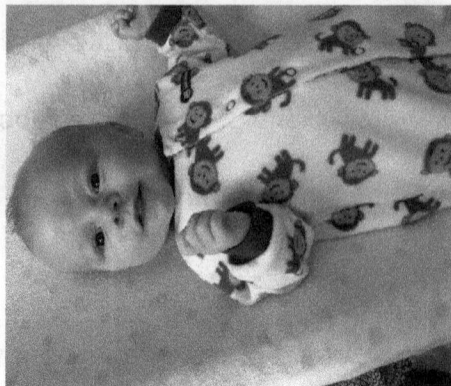

Mom: Tracy Standiford

\*\*\*

**For more testimonials, check out Doc Scharenberg's Youtube channel**

\*\*\*

## Acknowledgements

A special thanks to my daughter Jami for taking my scribbles and making them readable, also all the time and effort it took to help me make this dream a reality. And thanks to Ashley Shannon for her collaboration in the writing process. Jennifer, Melissa, Stephanie, and the office staff for their help and patience in this process.

I would like to thank all the parents of all the babies I have treated for their faith and confidence. Over the last forty years, I have had the privilege of caring for over a 1,000 babies who had the dreadful condition known as colic. Each of these babies have been affected to different degrees. Without them, it would have been impossible to research, learn, and create a technique that addresses baby's colic.

All of these babies and families have gone through much hardship, and it is my prayer that people be able to benefit from all the work that has gone into creating this technique. I hope that it will eventually prevent colic and, in turn, save babies, not only from their pain, but also from Shaken Baby Syndrome. Thousands of babies die every year from this condition, which is caused by the frustration of a caregiver.

I also want to thank my wife and children, as they have patiently and graciously allowed me to treat many of these babies on my days off, weekends, and holidays.

And a special thank you to my grandchildren who graciously shared their grandpa on many family occasions to treat these suffering babies. The hours of listening to crying babies have been hard, but the results have been gratifying. God has blessed me and my family.

# Sources

Chapter 1

1. "Understanding Colic---The Basics." Reviewed by Roy
   Benaroch. *Web MD,* 1 Mar. 2015. Web.

2. Hickey, Mary C. "The Tragedy of Shaken Baby Syndrome."
   *Parents Magazine.* November 2001. Web.

Chapter 2

1. Beck, Melinda. "Baby Crying? Doctors Say It May Be Acid-
   Reflux Disease." *The Wall Street Journal.* 22 July 2008. Web.

2. Barr, Ronald G., MD. "Colic and Crying Syndromes in Infants."
   *Pediatrics* 102.5 (Nov. 1998): 1282-286. Web.

Chapter 3

1. "Infantile Colic." *University of Maryland Medical Center.* 4 Aug.
   2014. Web.

2. Landau, Maryl Davids. "Alternative, Natural Medicine for
   Babies: Five drug-free cures for colds, colic, constipation, and
   more." *Parenting.* 2015. Web.

3. Perry, Rachel, et al. "Nutritional Supplements and Other
   Complementary Medicines for Infantile Colic: A Systematic

Review." *American Academy of Pediatrics.* Mar. 2011. Web.

4. O'Donovan, J. Crossan & Alden S. Bradstock, Jr. "The Failure of Conventional Drug Therapy in the Management of Infantile Colic." *Am J Dis Child* 133.10 (1 Oct. 1979): 999-1001. 2015. Web.

5. "Infants Simethicone." *WebMD.* 2015. Web.

6. "Everything you always wanted to know about the gut microbiota. . ." *Gut Microbiota Worldwatch.* 2016. Web.

7. "Understanding Probiotics." *Canadian Digestive Health Foundation.* 2016. Web.

8. Rhoads, J. Marc, et al. "Altered Fecal Microflora and Increased Fecal Calprotectin in Infants with Colic." *The Journal of Pediatrics* 155.6 (Dec. 2009): 823-28.e1. Web.

9. Savino, Francesco, et al. "Ghrelin and motilin concentration in Colicky Infants." *Acta Paediatr* 95.6 (Jun. 2006): 738-41. Web.

10. Chau, Kim, et al. "Probiotics for infantile colic: a randomized, double-blind placebo-controlled trial investigating Lactobacillus reuteri DSM 17938." *J Pediatr* 166.1 (Jan 2015): 74-78. Epub 23 Oct. 2014. Web.

11. Savino, Francesco, et al. "Lactobacillus reuteri (American Type Culture Collection Strain 55730) versus simethicone in the treatment of infantile colic: a prospective randomized study." *Pediatrics* 119.1 (Jan. 2007): e124-30. Web.

12. Petersen, Donald M., Jr. "The 37 Percent Solution." *Dynamic Chiropractic* 18.16 (24 July 2000). Web.

Chapter 4

1. "Newborn Reflexes." *What to Expect.* 2016. Web.

2. Torjesen, Ingrid. "Swaddling increases babies' risk of hip abnormalities." *BMJ.* 29 Oct. 2013. Web.

3. "AAP Expands Guidelines for Infant Sleep Safety and SIDS Risk Reduction." *American Academy of Pediatrics.* 18 Oct. 2011. Web.

4. Hughes, Sarah C., et al. "Infant Sleep Machines and Hazardous Sound Pressure Levels." *Pediatrics.* Feb. 2014. *American Academy of Pediatrics.* Web.

(Same information regarding study)

Landau, Elizabeth. "Sound machines for babies: Too loud? Too close?" *CNN.* 3 Mar. 2014. Web.

5. "Drowsy Driving Just As Dangerous As Drunk Driving: Study."

   *Huff Post Healthy Living.* 31 May 2012. Web.

6. Lawrence, Ruth A. & Robert M. Lawrence. *Breastfeeding: A*

   *Guide for the Medical Professionals.* Elsevier Health Sciences,

   13 Oct. 2015. E-book.

7. Used for this section: Karp, Harvey. *The Happiest Baby on the*

   *Block: The New Way to Calm Crying and Help Your Newborn*

   *Baby Sleep Longer.* NY: Batam Books, 2002. Print.

8. Esposito, Gianluca, et al. "Infant Calming Responses during

   Maternal Carrying in Humans and Mice." *Current Biology 23* (6

   May 2013): 739-45. Web.

9. Gray, Lisa, et al. "Skin-to-Skin Contact is Analgesic in Healthy

   Newborns." *Pediatrics* 105.1 (Jan. 2001): 1-6. Web.

10. Barr, Ronald, et al. "Carrying as colic 'therapy': A Randomized

    Controlled Trial." *Pediatrics* 87(5): 623-30. May 1991. Web.

Chapter 6

1. "Depression during and after pregnancy fact sheet." *Office of*

   *Women's Health, U.S. Department of Health and Human*

   *Services.* 16 July 2012. Web.

2. Bennett, Shoshana S. & Pec Indman. *Beyond the Blues: A Guide to Understanding and Treating Prenatal and Postpartum Depression.* San Jose, CA: Moodswings Press, 2003. Print. (p. 35)

Chapter 7

1. Hoeker, Jay L. "Infant and Toddler Health." *Web Md.* 2015. Web.

More reading on this chapter: "Your Digestive System and How it Works." *U.S. Department of Health and Human Services. NIH Publication*, 18 Sept. 2013. Web.

Chapter 8

1. Neifert, Marianne, M.D. *Dr. Mom's Guide to Breastfeeding.* NY: Plume-Penguin Group, 1998. Print. (p. 72-83, 222, & 273)

2. Spitzfaden, Laura. "Tongue-Tie and Lip-Tie." *Feed the Baby LLC.* 2012. Web.

3. Dessinger, Heather. "A Step-by-Step Guide to Checking for Tongue/Lip Ties." *Mommypotamus.* 2016. Web.

4. Genevieve. "How to Increase Milk Supply Naturally." *Mama Natural.* 2016. Web

5. Genevieve. "Oversupply: Tips for Engorgement and Making too much Milk." *Mama Natural.* Web.

6. Genevieve. "Overactive Letdown: Signs and Solutions for Baby and Momma."

A helpful resource with a list of studies on colic: Dewar, Gwen, PhD. *Parenting Science.* "Infantile Colic Research." 2015. Web.

**Treatment Goals and Motivations**

This document is for your record keeping. Feel free to copy for your own use.

What are your and your family's goals for treating your baby?

When you get discouraged, what will be your motivation?

What inspires you to treat your baby?

Who can be a source of encouragement to you while your baby is going through the colic treatment? How will you ensure he or she knows and understands what you will need?

How will you remember that patience is key?

Patient
Name_____DOB_____Date___/___/____

What would you consider your baby's percentage of **improvement** since starting treatment?

0% 5% 10% 15% 20% 25% 30% 35% 40% 45% 50% 55% 60% 65% 70% 75%

80% 85% 90% 95% 100%

When was the last **Bowel Movement**?


How many hours did he/she sleep total last night?

**Crying times** _____:_____ _____:_____ _____:_____ _____:_____

**Circle:**

**Spitting Up:**　　Mild　　　Moderate　　　Bad　　None

**Crying:**　　　　Mild　　　Moderate　　　Bad

　　　　　　　　For Pain　For Hunger　　Other

**Fussing:**　　　Mild　　　Moderate　　　Bad　　None

**Gassy:**　　　　Mild　　　Moderate　　　Bad　　None

**If Breastfeeding; have you had**: Fruits, Tomatoes, Rice, Nuts,

Broccoli, Cauliflower, Celery, Lettuce, Chocolate, Caffeine,

Cinnamon, Garlic, Onions, Peppers, Eggs, Beef, or Pork?

**Meal Examples**

|  | Breakfast | Lunch | Snack | Dinner |
|---|---|---|---|---|
| Day One | Cheerios with strawberries and milk. | Plain chicken sandwich with cheese. Carrots sticks on the side. | Cottage cheese with blueberries. | Plain turkey with peas and corn. |
| Day Two | Oatmeal with honey and fruit. | Turkey with melted cheese on a plain tortilla. | Baked apple slices with vanilla ice cream. | Plain pasta with grilled chicken, sautéed (in oil) carrots and green beans. |
| Day Three | Plain toast with vanilla yogurt and raspberries. | Baked potato with cheese, cottage cheese, and corn. | carrot sticks. | Shepherd's pie with ground turkey, corn, green beans, & mashed potatoes. |
| Day Four | Cheerios with blueberries and milk. | Homemade cheese pizza (omit the tomato paste and use tortilla for crust). | Vanilla yogurt with fruit. | Plain chicken with a baked potato and peas. |

| | | | | |
|---|---|---|---|---|
| Day Five | Oatmeal with honey and fruit. | Homemade chicken noodle soup with carrots and peas. (Omit any onions, celery, or other flavoring. Plain chicken broth is fine.) | Vanilla pudding with vanilla wafers. | Macaroni and cheese with grilled chicken and green beans. |
| Day Six | Plain toast with vanilla yogurt and pears. | Plain turkey sandwich with cheese. Carrot sticks on the side. | Vanilla ice cream with apple sauce. | Chicken and cheese tortilla with sour cream. |
| Day Seven | Cheerios with blackberries and milk. | Plain pasta with ground turkey and corn. | Cottage cheese with pineapple. | Ground turkey burger with cheese and a baked potato (sour cream, cheese, butter). |
| Day Eight | Oatmeal with honey and fruit. | Macaroni and cheese with green beans. | Cheese and plain crackers. | Plain turkey with sautéed potatoes, carrots, and peas. |
| Day Nine | Plain toast with vanilla yogurt and oranges. | Plain chicken with mashed potatoes and peas. | Grapes. | Plain turkey sandwich with cheese and carrot sticks on the side. |

| | | | | |
|---|---|---|---|---|
| Day Ten | Cheerios with strawberries and milk. | Plain chicken sandwich with cheese. Carrot sticks on the side. | Fruit smoothie with vanilla yogurt. | Crock Pot meal with cooked ground turkey on the bottom, potatoes and carrots on top. |

## Feeding Record

This document is for your record keeping. Feel free to copy for your own use.

| Date & Time | Breastfed or Bottle? | If bottle, how much given? | If breastfed, how long on each side? | Burped? | Spit up or projectile vomit? |
|---|---|---|---|---|---|
| | | | | | |
| | | | | | |
| | | | | | |
| | | | | | |
| | | | | | |
| | | | | | |
| | | | | | |
| | | | | | |
| | | | | | |
| | | | | | |
| | | | | | |
| | | | | | |
| | | | | | |
| | | | | | |
| | | | | | |
| | | | | | |
| | | | | | |

## About the Author

Dr. Dennis Scharenberg was born in 1948. He was injured at age seven in a horse accident. After the accident, he experienced various symptoms in his head and neck including pain, headaches, vision problems, tics, and tremors. All treatment failed to correct these problems until someone suggested chiropractic care. That's when progress began. He went for treatment for an extended period of time and was brought back to full health.

From this experience, he realized how valuable chiropractic care was. Even as a young person, this created a deep and sincere interest in becoming a chiropractic physician.

In 1973, Scharenberg graduated from Logan College of Chiropractic in St. Louis, Missouri. He raised his family in the small farming community of Hillsboro, Kansas, and practiced there for 35 years. Wanting to be near his children and grandchildren, he and his wife, Phyllis, decided to move to Wichita, Kansas, where Scharenberg is currently practicing, specializing in children and babies. He is certified in post graduate work in Sports and Recreation Injuries from

Los Angeles College of Chiropractic and post graduate studies of Idiopathic Scoliosis. He is a Fellow in Acupuncture Society of America and International Academy of Clinical Acupuncture.

During Scharenberg's career, he has done extensive research and created a specialized technique to address colic. He has treated over a 1,000 colic babies from all over the United States and various other countries. Along with this book, he has created educational videos on colic to teach parents all over the world how to treat their colicky babies.

Scharenberg has been a member of the Kansas Chiropractic Association since 1973. He has served on the board of directors for several years as secretary treasurer and vice president. He also served as president of the Kansas Chiropractic Foundation for many years. In 2006, Scharenberg was awarded "Doctor of the Year" by his peers in the Kansas Chiropractic Association.

Scharenberg has dedicated his entire life to helping people regain their health. His passion for helping babies has only increased with his experience, and he says he has no plans of retiring. He is affectionately known by his patients and staff as "Doc."